The Joyful Freedom Approach
to Cancer-Related Fatigue

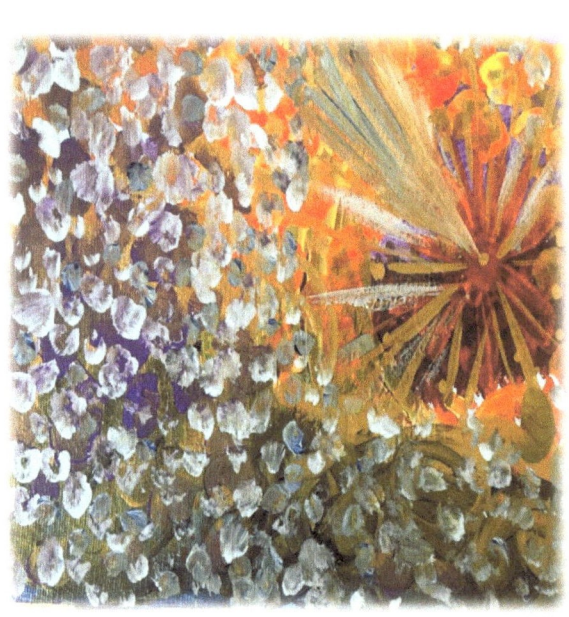

Marilynne N. Kirshbaum

The Joyful Freedom Approach to Cancer-Related Fatigue

Introducing an Energy-Creating Framework

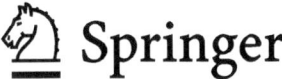 Springer

Marilynne N. Kirshbaum
Charles Darwin University
Darwin
NT
Australia

ISBN 978-3-030-76931-4   ISBN 978-3-030-76932-1   (eBook)
https://doi.org/10.1007/978-3-030-76932-1

This Springer imprint is published by the registered company Springer Nature Switzerland AG
The registered company address is: Gewerbestrasse 11, 6330 Cham, Switzerland

Dedicated to the little ones: Amelia, Mae and Emma

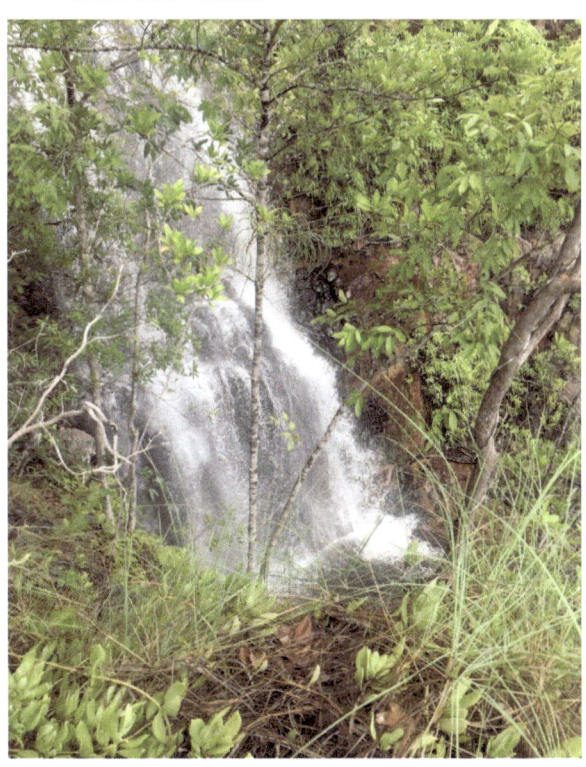

Tjaetaba Falls, Litchfield National Park
photo by Marilynne N. Kirshbaum

Acknowledgements

I wish to give thanks, from the depth of my heart to ...

The many amazing individuals whom I have met during my research who have trusted me with their stories, experiences and insights. Your faces, presence and words have carried me through, more than you will ever know;

Florence and Harry Kirshbaum, Esq., Martin Hartley Jackson, Nicola Young Jackson and Daniel Harry Jackman for their love and encouragement;

Springer Nature Publishers for providing me with the opportunity to write and be read widely;

Carey Vail and Laurence James Lucas for their beautiful 'out of this world' artwork;

The 'Dream Team' of the Breast Care Unit, Huddersfield Royal Infirmary, Huddersfield, UK: Richard Sainsbury, Valerie Walker, Rosemary Ainsworth, Alison Allen and incredible staff nurses;

Cheryl-lya Broadfoot, Professor Elizabeth Rosser, Professor Kärin Olson, Professor Karen Luker and Professor Kinta Beaver for their wise and patient mentorship; and Dr Gretchen Ellis for her continued inspiration and friendship.

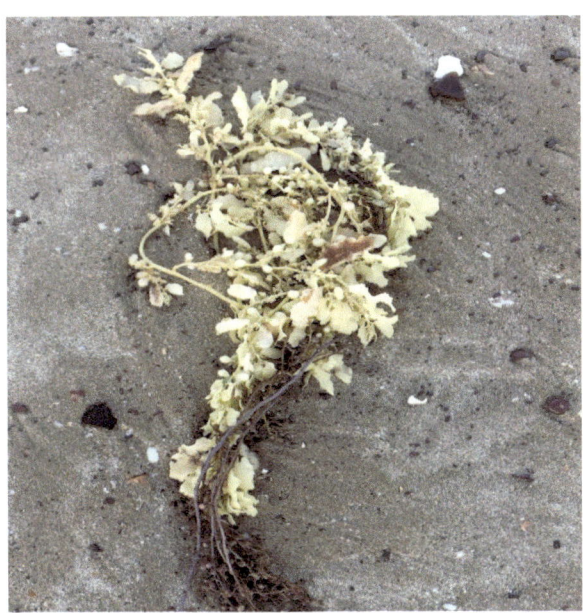

Seaweed on Casuarina Beach: photo by Marilynne N. Kirshbaum

Contents

Introduction

1.1 Background

It is 2020, an auspicious year and the dawn of a new decade that has been birthed amid worldwide upheaval. The world has witnessed unprecedented ravaging fires, devastating floods, political carnage, revolts of the masses and crumbling, corrupt institutions that have previously provided us with the firm foundations we thought were needed to progress through our precious lives. Then, there was the start of the COVID-19 pandemic, the severe economic consequences of lockdown and a worldwide call to confront racism spurred on by multiple incidences of senseless violence and racism in the United States. There is a feeling that these very real events are also symbolic representations of the intense change that is upon all of us.

Our humanness calls us forth to find a way to survive, somehow as the primitive dragonfly (Fig. 1.1). Through and despite the deep pain, despair, helplessness, anger and frustration in response to world events and the confinement of lockdown endured by millions, an activating sense of unified consciousness is emerging and with it, a realisation that we are all in this together. The most effective way out of this is surely to find better ways to help each other. The innate timidity and reserve in many of us needs to figure out how to shift into courageousness—to take action and not hold back any longer.

Hence begins this book on energy and personal well-being—because as a healthcare professional, counsellor, hypnotherapist, researcher, educator and spiritual guide, it is what I can offer now. From my perspective, the way to navigate the future successfully lays in tapping into the life force that is available to us throughout our day-to-day lives. Energy is the force and quality that propels, nourishes and sustains our body and mind 24 hours a day. Where does the energy come from? Where does it go? How do we use it? and How can we get more of it to enable us to thrive and not sink into a spiral of hopelessness, exhaustion and misery?

I have spent many years contemplating, researching and teaching the multidimensional parts of the enigmatic subject of cancer-related fatigue and have learnt

© Springer Nature Switzerland AG 2021   1
M. N. Kirshbaum, *The Joyful Freedom Approach to Cancer-Related Fatigue*,
https://doi.org/10.1007/978-3-030-76932-1_1

Fig. 1.1 Dragonfly on
bird of paradise photo by
Marilynne N Kirshbaum

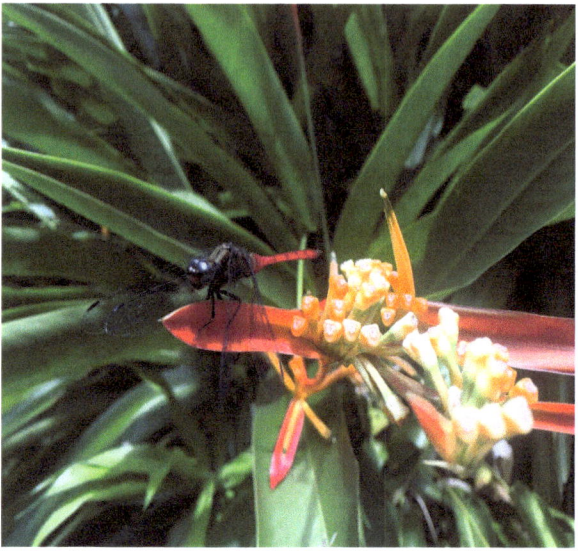

quite a bit. There are parts of the grand puzzle that are known and are well evidenced in the research literature, but there are also many under-researched aspects that may never ever be understood sufficiently to become acceptable, accessible or affordable to those in most need.

This book speaks to healthcare professionals and other interested readers who are intrigued by the existence of an energy-creating framework. My long-standing fascination and study of well-being and specifically cancer-related fatigue has been inspired firsthand by spending lots of time with people who have experienced cancer. As a nurse and subsequent researcher, I witnessed the deleterious effects of cancer and its treatment on the kindest, most cherished, intelligent, sensitive, graceful, kind, outrageous, hilarious, generous, despairing, angry, obnoxious and frightened cohort of humanity. The generosity and honesty of patients, clients and research participants enabled me to capture the details of how cancer and the fatigue associated with the illness impacted upon their thoughts, emotions, relationships and actions. The qualitative, empirical and experiential research undertaken in stages for over 35 years has led me to develop an individualised lifelong self-care program that is life-affirming and energising!

My interest in energetic health and well-being is longstanding, personal and profound. I have immersed myself in this broad and diverse area throughout my lifetime. I have uncovered vast knowledge, accessed research-based resources and explored many modalities of energy medicine experientially. After so many years as a professional nurse, I remain fascinated and even exuberant as I continue to learn, experience, evaluate and report upon the potential of a growing number of therapeutic approaches and strategies used to reduce the debilitating effects of extreme tiredness, lethargy and fatigue.

My excitement and motivation come from knowing that there is an infinite amount of available energy that surrounds us, right now. It is up to us as healthcare professionals and human beings to tap into this vast reservoir of energetic and healing 'cosmic gold dust' that has the potential to fortify the physical, mental, emotional and spiritual dimensions of health for ourselves and fellow travellers who share this planet in this space and time with us today.

Energy has always fascinated me. Everything is made up of energy, and it exists for us to use all the time! According to my memory of what I was taught in school, I learned about the different forms of energy: kinetic/potential, mechanical, chemical and convection. When I investigated the topic today, I see that there is also thermal, nuclear, electromagnetic, sonic, gravitational and ionizing energy (Helmenstine 2020). It is actually very exciting to know because through my research and work in healing energy, there is so much that has not been explained. I am convinced that many of the answers to the as yet unexplained or substantiated modes of treatment or therapies will be found in the physical sciences. There is still so much that we as humans beings do not understand. So much of what we do is unsubstantiated, and this includes the 'accepted' protocols and procedures found in modern acute-care hospitals. As a nursing student, we were encouraged to question and then search the research literature for an explanation—but so often the evidence was non-existent or very weak.

This book attempts to gather what is known about cancer-related fatigue from credible and evidence-based research and to provide some awareness of the less investigated modes of intervention and treatment. I have a vision of integrating many forms of knowledge and practice of which I have tried to present to the readers of this book. I will be leading you through a personal narrative of my explorations that culminate in the last chapter as a preliminary version of the Joyful Freedom Approach for Energy Restoration. Readers may find the words that I use surrounding energy such as being a 'life-force' a bit whimsical, but it is my way of bridging the positivist evidence with the infinite unknown that I honestly view as magical and part of the cosmic realms, yet to be revealed. Please rest assured that my vision is grounded in nursing research and clinical oncology practice, although I remain open to understanding and knowledge without any boundaries—it is a life quest. I feel quite honoured to be able to present a lifetime of work and ponderings to you.

1.2 The Joyful Freedom Approach

The Joyful Freedom Approach emerged from years of observation in mainly oncology nursing practice, rigourous concept-based nursing research, continuous personal exploration and a fair measure of creative flow involving intuition, the arts, connection to nature and sexual life-force explorations.

The approach has been developed through a series of research studies inspired initially by women who had breast cancer and were troubled by ongoing cancer-related fatigue. This body of research, which includes a PhD study in Nursing and numerous articles published in peer-reviewed academic journals, has culminated in identifying five attributes of energy restorative activities; these are represented in the Energy Restoration Framework (Table 9.1).

The Joyful Freedom Approach is not passive. It is:

- active, subjective, empowering, self-motivating, expansive, practical, objective-based, self-managed, freedom enhancing and energy-generating;
- focused on observing one's own daily activities, lifestyle choices and goals;
- evidenced-based and developed from research with people who have cancer and/or palliative care conditions;
- adaptable, life-affirming and ultimately energy creating, fun and joyful;
- problem-based as a way to identify an issue, concern or barrier to moving forward to reveal a more fulfiling, comfortable, energised, happy way of living in the now—day to day;
- a gentle, compassionate and individual approach that accelerates the ability to find energetic balance, strengthen decision-making, address helplessness and promote beneficial transformation into a renewed vision of self or more practically address a physical, emotional, cognitive or spiritual problem.

There will not be any 'no-go areas' because everything that comes into a person's mind, world or informational platform should be viewed as something that has the potential for being energy creating. If it holds interest and fascinates a person, even it if dismissed by others as being silly, boring or 'crackers', could still have an energy-creating effect or outcome.

The five attributes of energy creation and sustainability are PECAN: *Purposeful, Expanding, Connecting/Belonging, Awe-inspiring* and *Nourishing* They represent infinite types of activities that connect directly to what one truly wants to do. Some would say it encourages delving deep into one's heart space or into their soul to entice an individual's joy to emerge. Concurrently, the framework acknowledges the importance of bringing awareness to the blocks and barriers that limit the full positive, joyful expression of a person's emotional, physical and cognitive self.

The framework uses the attributes conceptually as they represent more than just a word or term, but each can be explored from different perspectives and studied deeply, for each will lead to creative modes and programs for lifelong self-care and management. The framework is intended to be used practicaly as a care plan or action plan and is flexible and adaptable for use by a healthcare practitioner, cancer patient/client and really anyone who is interested in benefiting from a boost of energy and subtle lifestyle transformation.

I have been using my own recent experience of recovery from heart surgery on top of some common 'sources of energy zapping', such as overwhelm of work, social expectations, relationship choices and travel. Although I have not experienced cancer, I have still gained so much from experiential development and experimentation surrounding energy restoration. It has been an interesting and fortifying journey.

The attributes (PECAN) act as headings for self-reflection and analysis, action planning and intentional integration into an individual's recovery phase of life following illness, trauma and beyond. Moreover, as the reader will discover, the Framework has a universal appeal to all of us who at times feel preoccupied with non-specific anxieties and worries or feel like we have well and truly 'lost the plot' to our lives. I hope you will find something useful within these pages.

1.3   Overview

The book, The Joyful Freedom Approach to Cancer-related Fatigue: Introducing an Energy-creating Framework, is organised into three parts and subdivided into chapters. Part One contains the chapters of: The Inspiration, The Challenge and the Resolution. These first chapters offer the reader a gateway to the Joyful Freedom Approach starting with a narrative that starts from my time at university studying nursing and discovering energy fields, through to the foundations and detail surrounding evidence-based research on cancer-related fatigue and possible interventions. Part Two consists of chapters that serve to place the energy-creating framework in context: Philosophy and Theory, Evidence for Change and Research in Practice. Here, the influential Attention Restorative Theory of Professor Stephen Kaplan, an environmental psychologist, is introduced. The discussion then progresses onto the adaptation of Kaplan's theory to the cancer care and illness context. Part Three provides an overview and representation of The Energy Restoration Framework leading to the emergence of the Joyful Freedom Approach.

This book is aimed at healthcare practitioners who, in the course of their interactions with clients and patients, find themselves in the position of counselling people through distressful life events. This would include nurses, occupational therapists, social workers, mental health practitioners and medical doctors who work with individuals who are recovering not only from cancer but also from illnesses or surgery and are interested in helping their clients regain control and navigate their own path to wellness. The book offers practitioners an evidence-based approach that is versatile and adaptable to meet the needs of a varied range of clients.

Reference

Helmenstine AM. 10 types of energy and examples. ThoughtCo; 2020. https://www.thoughtco.com/main-energy-forms-and-examples-609254. Accessed 14 April 21. ·

The Inspiration: Energy Fields and the Science of Unitary Beings

2

2.1   From the Beginning

We are birthed and then go off to live our lives along some sort of path. This is our own unique and precious *Journey of Life* that truly holds so much potential (Fig. 2.1). Human history and our collective culture exist to inform and direct us along the

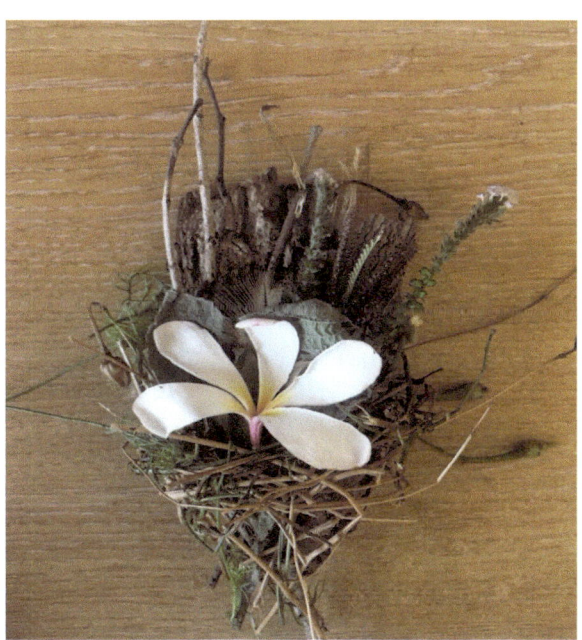

Fig. 2.1 An offering to the Journey of Life by Marilynne N. Kirshbaum

way, sometimes without us being aware. The social norms of our local communities and countries may at times be oppressive and painfully constricting, yet they play important roles that are inevitable and unavoidable. Still, there is value and power in the belief that there may well be unexplored opportunities to seek, discover and immerse ourselves in as we find meaningful pursuits that nourish, inspire, heal, inform, fascinate, love and care for others. Sometimes, the road to find our own *life purpose* is obvious, clear, defined, smooth and full of abundance. Sometimes the journey presents endless tragedy, hardship and despair.

For most of us, our life flow is variable; we have good times and not-so-good times that prompt us to put in more effort and push ourselves through whatever obstacles block our way. Some of us adopt strategies to create more focus and efficiency while also welcoming in creativity to get ourselves back on track, or so we think. At other times, lethargy, stagnation, paralysis, helplessness and hopelessness take centre stage. Here, there are two stark choices: wait it out or do something about it.

Throughout my life so far, I have realised that although it is a great idea to have both long- and short-range plans, one's *life journey* has a way of weaving a path of its own. It is not really about having a plan. It is more about figuring out how you are going to navigate through the turbulent or sluggish phases. This 'how' is derived directly from our values, beliefs and attitudes, which determine our behaviours. Our parents started us off by giving us life and had the responsibility of being our first nurturers and providers of nourishment. Then, for the majority of us, our teachers and their assistants in schools set out to inculcate rules and behaviours surrounding how to exist with others and adhere to the status quo. At this early stage, we engaged in the basics of self-awareness and accountability. In tandem with the physical and cognitive developments that are observed and noted as milestones, our personalities and talents began to show. In safe, stimulating and loving environments, these same personalities and talents can begin to blossom and flourish spontaneously and fully. There can be such delight in witnessing the emergence of a young person's character and charms through unobstructed expression, through to an older child and adult; a complete and self-actualised human being who has an abundance of confidence, curiosity, joy and sense of belonging. Let us take this in and pause for a moment. The same qualities can also be called upon to help us all through difficult times—but we need to find a way to develop, remember and access helpful qualities and actions.

You are invited to take a deep breath and just pause for a little while (Fig. 2.2).

Fig. 2.2 Delicate Top End
Northern Territory flower
photo by Marilynne
N. Kirshbaum

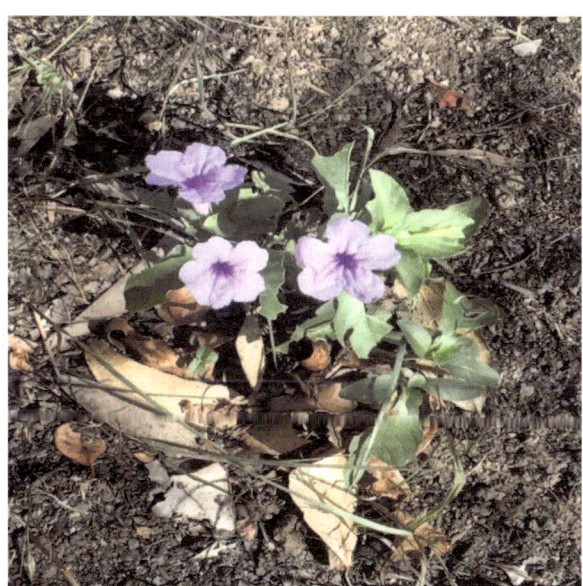

2.2   Life-Force Energy

This unashamedly raw and bright visual (Fig. 2.3) is positioned here to infuse life-affirming golden light into this early chapter on my background as an ardent and enthusiastic optimist who has spent her life developing an enlivening programme of self-care for emotional and physical recovery called '*The Joyful Freedom Approach*'. My story begins at this juncture, as I take you on a personal and scholarly journey through the significant signposts of an academic and professional life that draws from a long-standing fascination with the infinite and universal life-force energy that surrounds and exists within us.

I have always been fascinated by the diversity of people and their personal stories. Self-biography is a technique that I use in counselling to encourage a person to view their life objectively. This usually pulls out interesting and sometimes challenging insights into troubling issues and connections that might not have been identified previously. With the support of a counsellor as a guide, a troubling event or memory can be looked at closely and explored.

I am usually a cheerful and enthusiastic person, although I started out as being a rather shy only-child of two quite serious, devoted and hard-working mature adults

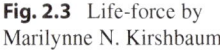

Fig. 2.3 Life-force by
Marilynne N. Kirshbaum

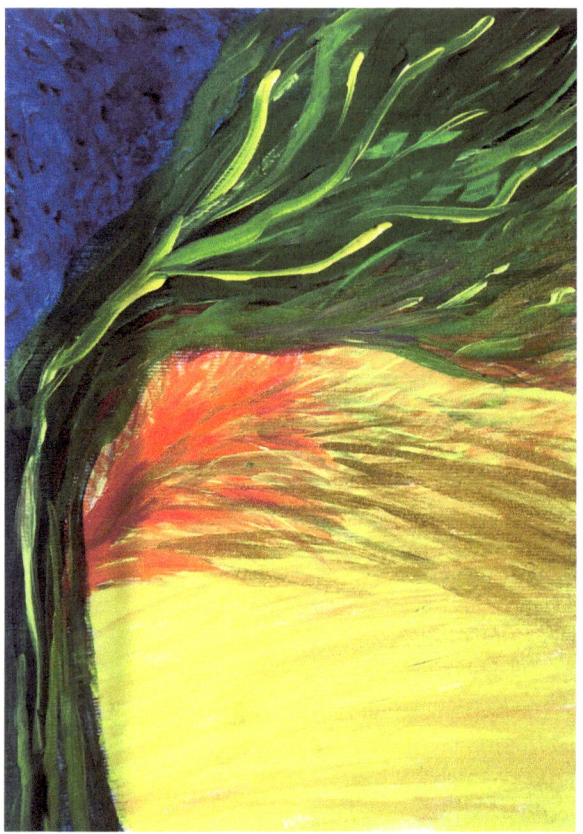

who provided me with an enriched home environment on the edge of Harlem in New York City. Everyone will have their own childhood memories. For most of us, these memories are infused with both happy and sad times, and some of us will have had to face adversity and damaging trauma of some kind. I view my childhood as being quite privileged although I have become an expert in blocking out much of the pain and hardship that I have experienced and can remember, if I try hard enough. I spent lots of time on a Caribbean Island in the West Indies way back in the 1960s, swimming in the clear, warm sea and playing in perfect sized waves to the soundtrack of steel drums and Reggae. Only children often spend lots of time on their own. I was encouraged to entertain myself by drawing and colouring, dancing and reading. I used my imagination and creativity often. I drew lots of trees—I remember that—I was always fascinated by trees, particularly weeping willows, and the way the light reflected from their sleepy, swaying and dancing leaves. The light and movement held a special quality for me, but it was hard to explain this to grown-ups. I did not have the right words, but I could express it in dance and sometimes in my abstract scribbles. There was movement, energy and something that existed that could not be touched, held or photographed. Now I call it life-force energy and I know that it is universal and infinite—it holds the key to self-healing—if only … If only people would allow themselves to open up their senses sufficiently to feel it, respected it and use it for their own benefit.

And so, I will begin to explain my interpretation of life-force energy. This might sound a bit 'new age' and at odds with the evidenced-based scientific paradigm that I present, but one does not and should not negate the other unless there is clear proof of disproof. My approach here, as in life, is to remain open and receptive to all possibilities and devote myself to exploration, discovery, understanding and then evaluation because we need to know what kinds of interventions and approaches to fatigue are effective and also why. I will be taking you through the research process of questioning and gathering evidence, but this will be in a non-conventional manner. My intention is to uncover unique perspectives and attempt to make useful linkages to stimulate the thought processes of practitioners and researchers to use as they see fit.

We are vessels of flowing, cosmic, emotional, mental, vibrating, pulsating, heat-producing, bright, magnetic, biochemical, sensual, sexual and alchemic energy. The life-force energy that flows through us is naturally abundant and healing. It is up to us to acknowledge, feel, observe and move it around to serve our basic and deeper needs and desires. This is my personal view that has been influenced by mainstream science available to me from educational institutions in the United States and United Kingdom, integrated into my younger self's observations, evidenced by internationally accepted empirical research and amplified by the increasingly credible sources of person-centred, subjective evidence.

2.3   The Science of Life

I have attended quite a few births, most recently welcoming three granddaughters into this world. I have observed the miraculous events through the eyes and intuitive awareness of the Grand-Ma, as I like to be called. At birth, there is lots of wriggling and some crying as the newborn leaves the physical cocoon of warmth and safety of the womb. Their little heart beats in response to an electro-chemical signal of the pacemaker; the newly initiated lungs begin to expand with the gaseous mixture of nitrogen and oxygen that flows through and nourishes the billions of cells in their tiny bodies. It is such a whopping physical moment accompanied by a full range of off-the-scale emotions that run wild in parallel. Then, once we know all seems okay or at least stable, we can settle down, rest and begin to adjust to the reality of a new little being who has joined this magnificent and crazy world.

From conception, and some would say even before that, our beginnings are characterised by a process of energy generation, flow and intricate exchanges between chemical elements, molecules, compounds and their associated ions that cause the reactions. The physical body can take in food and amazingly, break it down and distribute its parts in the form of nutrients and by products of reactions, enzymes and hormones to where it is needed. This ebb and flow of the silent biochemical and magnetic energy within us is continuous and functions miraculously in synchronicity and with resonance with hundreds of other simultaneous processes. This represents the foundational physical generators for life-force energy.

2.4   Systems Theory

The wonder of life is present throughout every moment of each day until the heartbeat stops, blood ceases to flow and nourish, and our body's organs cease to function. We die while others mourn our passing. However, what about the gap between life and death? It is complicated. One approach to describe and begin to understand how the puzzle of life is arranged is to acknowledge the history of philosophy and science. The early philosophers pondered life and humanity's existence. The early scientists took their observations of the natural world and began to explain what they saw systematically. Hippocrates wrote about health as being dependent on achieving a state of equilibrium of internal processes within the body and mind that involved living in harmony with the external environment. There is a hint of holistic and naturistic perspectives here. However, it appeared to have been lost or rather re-interpreted as the mechanistic, mind–body dualism of modern medical science emerged. Specialisms of body parts and physical and biological functions came into being, and health problems were treated in isolation, for example by a cardiologist, neurologist or psychiatrist.

While this was developing, Florence Nightingale, and those who were influenced by her revolutionary evidence-based practices, demonstrated the important role of the environment in both health and illness. This was cutting-edge thinking from a Western perspective. Our humanness was on the verge of being recognised seriously. The problem was not merely with the malfunctioning or infected body part but the way the human body, mind and spirit responded to an alteration. This response reflects the way the body takes action as an organised system orchestrating the various dynamic and interrelated parts. It is about the intricate relationships between the parts of the body—an acknowledgement of Systems Theory.

As a university student of the late 1970s and 1980s, my fascination with nature and humanity was encouraged through the study of psychology, anthropology and nursing. First, I studied psychology, which was interesting and followed on from an elective that took in high school, but at the university level, it seemed limited and quite stagnant in the way it was presented at the time. So, I transferred to a nursing course. The appeal was its breadth of scope; really, anything to do with people and health, and it was also quite practical in terms of getting a professional job straight after graduation as a registered nurse. I did much of the prerequisite science and social science units/modules at Boston University, gave lots of my attention toward medical and physical anthropology, which I adored, but I was first exposed to the art and science of nursing that I embraced so fully while I was at New York University (NYU) studying Nursing and Anthropology. This is when I began to learn about Systems Theory and the intricate interdependent relationships that existed between the parts of the body and mind—and I was blown away!

2.5   Energy Fields and the Science of Unitary Human Beings

Martha E. Rogers, previous Head of the Division of Nursing Education at NYU, and her visionary Science of Unitary Human Beings inspired me along the path and practice of nursing as an art and science, all those many years ago. Her scholarly and original conceptualisations set out in her *Science of Unitary Beings* (Rogers 1970) engaged me fully in becoming a registered nurse.

This was in the early 1980s when New York City was at one of the lowest points in its history. The city was bankrupt, lawless and dangerous. Deaths from violent crimes reached 2,500 per year. As a nursing student based in Greenwich Village, the emerging public health challenges of a crack-cocaine epidemic and the early effects of the then untreatable, HIV/AIDS were apparent and on display. The vigilante group called the *Guardian Angels* patrolled the subways, protecting the good citizens of the 'Greatest City in the World'—then.

I had recently returned to New York after attending university in Boston, Massacheusetts just five hours away by train. But in December 1980, life had thrown me a curveball. My father had a severe brain haemorrhage days before I was due to return home for the Christmas break and died after two weeks in a coma. This was the same week when John Lennon was shot and killed, not more than a mile from where I grew up. In the weeks that followed, a life-changing decision was made. I would return to New York and stay with my grieving mother and continue my studies at NYU. This was a hugely significant event for me.

Emeritus Professor [Guru] Martha E. Rogers inspired me like no one else. She wrote about the history of science, shifting paradigms, Systems Theory, energy fields, space-time as the fourth dimension, astral projections, nursing research and about highly abstract theoretical principles such as *integrality, helicy* and *resonancy* all in relation to the human being as a patient and as a human energy field. I read *An Introduction to the Theoretical Basis of Nursing* (Rogers 1970) with complete relish, several times. I was recognised academically and was commended for being a kind, caring and functionally efficient nursing student while also able to integrate and apply Rogers' principles to practical tasks as a nursing student with living patients. This was a joy for me—I really loved reading about energy fields and physics and the transcendent properties of energy waves and what was viewed as matter. It was emancipating to be a pioneer of a novel approach within a highly traditional, service-oriented 'call to service' of nursing that was now on the cusp of transforming into a true profession, along with its own research base.

Rogers was a visionary but not in the new-age or spiritual sense. She was a scientist—a nurse scientist who was able to think deeply and write with sufficient skill to influence academics to base an entire nursing program around her highly abstract elucidations. The abstractions were not comprehensible or appealing to the masses. However, a strength was that with a bit of concentration and acceptance, the theoretical statements, paradigm shift, principles and propositions all provided an intriguing structure and could, with some imagination and creativity, be applied to direct nursing practice, education and research.

2.6   Rogers' Conceptual Framework and Application

Now, as I look back and revisit Rogers' writing, I see how much of her work in the last century has been embedded in my view of nursing, health and understanding the world around me. Personally, I experienced an enigmatic 'spark' characterised by intellectual expansion, fascination, awe and wonder, which funnily enough will re-emerge later in this book as core concepts of energy restoration.

All this fuelled my interest in reading and learning as much as I could. I believed that nursing needed a holistic, intelligent and inspiring approach that would be able to address the needs of an ageing population with increasing complexity and multiple chronic comobidities. And that was back then—we are now making our way through the 2020s—and there is still reason to call Martha in—so here she is at the start—within this book on introducing a framework for energy restoration. Please note that much of what you will read here will be new and use unfamiliar terminology. I would encourage you to be open to different ways of thinking and take in what you can as the chapters unfold before you. Some parts of your brain may be sparked and enlivened in the process. I was driven to understand every aspect of her theory and took great delight in reading about the history of knowledge and different types of theory and philosophical frameworks that scholars have developed through the ages to make sense of the world.

When it came to understanding how we address illness, promote wellness and care for people based upon the knowledge that was tested through research, I was completely hooked on this kind of nursing—nursing for the new age—and this was 1981.

2.7   What Was So Special About Martha?

Nursing is a humanistic science dedicated to compassionate concern for maintaining and promoting health, preventing illness and caring for and rehabilitating the sick and disabled. Man*, whom nursing strives to serve, is a unified whole, a synergistic system, who cannot be explained by knowledge of his [their] parts. Sweeping changes taking place throughout the world emphasize life's creativity and challenge the most visionary to foretell the days ahead. The goals of achieving human health and welfare have taken on undreamed-of dimensions as man's earth-bound past merges with his space-directed future. (Rogers 1970, vii) *Man = Humanity

These words from the Foreword of Martha E. Rogers' *An Introduction to the Theoretical Basis of Nursing* (Rogers 1970) merged the altruistic and service aspects of nursing with the cosmic, pan-dimensional (beyond multi-dimensionality) and intergalactic perspective that inspired forward-thinking nurses from a long-forgotten era.

Martha's visionary articulations of professional nursing included the rise of modern science from the Stone Age, through ancient civilisations to modern times. Her vast and intoxicating account of history firmly planted nursing in its rightful place within science and philosophy.

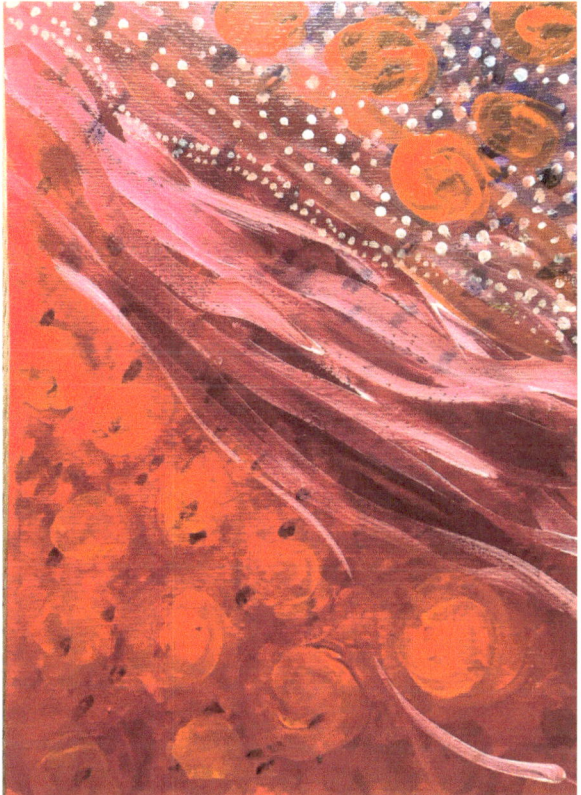

Fig. 2.4   Red River of Life by Marilynne N. Kirshbaum

Rogers identified and critically reviewed the extreme prevalence of the mechanistic view of the twentieth century, where humankind's roles and routines were segmented into different parts, namely the biological, physical, psychological, social and spiritual; each viewed as a 'function' with its own boundaries, limits and subjective research studies emanating from different disciplines.

In stark contrast, Rogers presented a then quite revolutionary exploratory perspective of humanity as a 'unified phenomenon' that had essence and function that was more than and different from the sum of its parts, that is, a systems approach.

Rogers wrote that all great thinkers and creatives of the current age (1960s and 70s) were faced with developing a new cosmology because old, previously accepted and followed presumptions that characterised medical practice were no longer adequate to build the future of the emergent Science of Nursing. In the next section, I will present the cornerstones of Rogers' theoretical explorations, principles and resultant conceptual model for nursing practice. A visual representation called *Red River of Life* appears in Fig. 2.4. I expect you will be struck at how contemporary her vision was with New-Age terminology of the 2020s.

2.8   The Theoretical Basis of Nursing According to Martha E. Rogers

Martha was not an 'airhead' or New Age Traveller; she was a scholar, philosopher, nurse scientist and theorist who went on to develop a grand conceptual theory for understanding humankind in its entirety, in its fullest complexity that has addressed the now prevalent acceptance of our multidimensional/pan-dimensional and unified energy fields. She was ahead of her time in declaring that the mechanistic way of viewing our social, political, physical, psychological and spiritual domains of life in isolation was ineffective and detrimental to our health and well-being, whereas taking a 'Living Systems' approach solidly rooted in systems theory made sense to a world where its inhabitants are dynamic, complex and in constant need of compassionate research-based care.

The foundation of *The Science of Unitary Human Beings*, best understood as a conceptual framework, consists of five assumptions (postulates), four (critical) elements or concepts and three overarching principles (fundamental guides to the practice of nursing). There have been several updates and developments over the years, but for now, I wish to lay out the basics as clearly as I can. Please note 'Man' denotes 'Humanity' and Martha most definitely included 'Woman'; 'Human being' was therefore used in the academic discourse that followed.

2.8.1   The Basic Assumptions

1. Man [human being] is a unified whole possessing its own integrity and manifesting characteristics that are more than and different from the sum of its parts (Rogers 1970, p. 47). [Wholeness]
   Here we begin with a major paradigm shift away from the mechanistic ways of traditional medical care. This assumption lays the foundation to holistic nursing care and just about all complementary therapies, where the person is viewed and accepted as a unique entity, comprising physical parts that function together, but also emotions, memories and individual character.
2. Man [human being] and environment are continuously exchanging matter and energy with one another (Rogers 1970, p.54) [Openness]
   The existence of a permeable boundary surrounding our physical, emotional and spiritual bodies is introduced here, which implies that we are affected by our surroundings. The environment here includes all living things and the other stimuli, for example smell, light, sound and vibration that surround the person. There is an energy field that is open, dynamic and responsive to the entire universe.
3. The life process evolves irreversibly along a space-time continuum (Rogers 1970, p. 59). [Unidirectionality]
   This assumption recognises that each life moves forward from birth to death. We increase in complexity as we age and advance. We do not go backwards or regress. This is quite profound and forward-thinking when we consider how we view older people and their inevitable changes both

externally (appearance) and internally (increased 'wear and tear' combined with increased morbidity).

4. *Pattern and organisation identify man* [human beings] and reflect his [their] innovative wholeness (Rogers 1970, p. 65). [Pattern and Organisation]

   Following on from the previous assumption that emphasises unidirectionality, Martha goes a step further and states that the way we move forward is ordered and not chaotic, nor determined by chance. The process is directly influenced by the way the person, as an energy field, interacts with their environment. One way to observe fluctuations is through technologies such as high-voltage Kirlian photography that can be used to capture the phenomenon of electrical coronal discharges i.e. auras.

5. Man [human being] is characterised by the capacity for abstraction and imagery, language and thought, sensation and emotion. (Rogers 1970, p. 73). [Sentience and Thought]

   The final assumption reminds us of our higher level qualities that distinguish human beings from other living creatures. No other life form that we know of ponders its existence or future or is so rooted in ritual, art or philosophy. Other living beings may have well-developed senses, some far exceeding ours, but as far as we know, the depth and scope of their abilities do not include abstract interpretation, that is, our thoughts are entwined with our feelings and emotions; this has implications for intelligent and holistic nursing care. There is also the integration of advanced language, evolution and transcendence to consider under this assumption.

2.8.2   The Elements

The Science of Unitary Human Beings integrates four key elements that act as concepts and were best defined well after Rogers' original work: *Energy fields, Open systems, Pattern* and *Pandimensionality* (Rogers 1986, 1991). Very briefly, Rogers viewed the energy field as the 'fundamental unit of living and non-living' (Rogers 1986)—it contained, encompassed and acted as 'the whole'. There were only two energy fields to consider: (1) the human energy field (the person) and (2) the environment energy field, which included everything else. *Open systems* explain the way the energy fields continuously reacted to each other—they were not rigid membranes. *Patterns* here are quite unique; they are perceived abstractly [and not quite fully explained] as a single wave (Rogers 1986). *Pan-dimensionality* goes beyond our three-dimensional perceptions and deliberately encourages us to not just consider but accept and integrate the 'unexplainable' phenomena of the time, for example astral projection, spiritual events, déjà vu and the supernatural into nursing care (Biley 1995). This was a time before scientists became aware of quantum physics, quarks and existence of black holes in the universe. Indeed, these are abstract discoveries that remain incomprehensible to the general public but are available nevertheless to ponder and perhaps understand for those with the appropriate aptitude and foundational knowledge.

2.8.3   The Principles of Homeodynamics

Rogers' offering to nursing was never truly considered to be a theory, but rather an abstract system; a new paradigm for nursing called nursing science. There were no testable hypotheses formulated; however, her work sparked a substantial following, primarily in North America, from her base at New York University—where I studied nursing in a program that integrated Rogerian Science into every aspect of teaching, assessment and applied nursing practice. Nursing scholars studying for higher degrees were inspired to pick up on different aspects of Roger's conceptual system, inspired to advance and conduct ground-breaking research and further develop practice and education that followed the five assumptions, leading to the formulation of new and expanded theories of nursing.

The operationalisation of Rogers' framework to clinical practice was initiated through the Principles of Homeodynamics, which have been a bit 'dynamic' over the years through ongoing refinements. They were introduced in Rogers' first book as symbolic, provisional, hypothetical generalizations and theories derived 'from the imaginative synthesis of available data' (Rogers 1970, p. 95). In effect, the principles were postulates on the constantly changing and exchanging nature of the human and environmental energy fields, described as a homeodynamic life process, that required testing and confirmation. They still do. An overview of the principles of *Integrality, Helicy* and *Resonancy* follows, accompanied by a few examples to provide an indication of how they can be used to influence direct patient care.

At the foundation is *Integrality*. First, one needs to understand the view that the human body is a porous energy field that exists continuously with and is integral to the surrounding environment. They are both open systems, but the exchange is simultaneous—one field does not 'affect' the other, they are a part of one another. However, if a change is initiated, for example, a nurse opens a window to bring in some fresh air or plays some music, the human and environmental fields may both benefit from that action.

Helicy 'connotes that the life process evolves unidirectionally in sequential stages along a curve which does not lie in a plane' (Rogers 1970, p. 99). This principle notes that we are always moving forward to reach our goals, even if we have not articulated our own ones yet. We have the propensity to progress forward in some way; that is our nature, but the path is not straight. We exist in space-time, which has a spiral shape, evolving creatively and unpredictably through our innovations and experiences. Life is not about reaching equilibrium or homeostasis—that would be viewed as being stagnant. *Helicy* can be such a life affirming principle, if comprehended and applied fully, as it acknowledges the existence and value of every life event. We learn, develop and progress from every aspect of our lives, even if it feels stagnant or stuck.

Through *Resonancy*, the quality of our forward movement is expressed as moving in waves, from low frequency to higher frequencies. 'The life process in Man [Humanity] is a symphony of rhythmical vibrations oscillating at various frequencies' (Rogers 1970, p. 101). Here it is explained that so much of what defines us as humans: our perceptions, emotions, auras and our universe fluctuate as light,

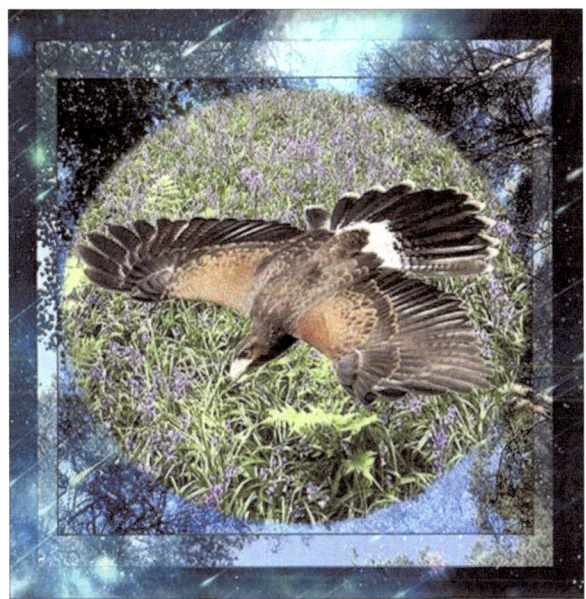

Fig. 2.5   Eagle by Carey Vail

sound and gravity. All exist and flow like waves. To promote health and healing, nurses are encouraged to support the natural pattern and organisation of the individual sensitively and intelligently. The focus of care is on providing support for the integrity of the human energy field as it changes through re-patterning. Through this lens of the Rogerian trained nurse, the person is always changing, and it is the nurse's role to support the person through it. For example, think of the person recovering from surgery, any surgery. The nurse is there to assess and respond to all aspects of recovery and towards improved wellness.

Martha Rogers has provided the inspiration that was made available to me at a critical time in my life, to embrace nursing and commit to a path that stimulated my mind to seek out knowledge for the benefit of humanity. The Eagle (Fig. 2.5) represents the value of taking a view of the world from high in the sky, far above life on Earth, but still very much a part of this world. Rogers' framework has provided a background to what will now unfold in relation to cancer-related fatigue.

References

Biley FC. Providing a conceptual framework for practice (Chapter Three). In: Sayre-Adams J, Wright S, editors. The theory and practice of therapeutic touch. Edinburgh: Churchill Livingston; 1995.

Rogers ME. An introduction to the theoretical basis of nursing. Philadelphia: F A Davies; 1970.

Rogers ME. Science of unitary human beings. In Malinski V M (Ed) Explorations on Martha Rogers' science of human beings. New York: National League for Nursing; 1986.

Rogers ME. Glossary Rogerian Nursing Science News. 1991;4(2):6–7.

3

3.1 Introduction

The abstract vibrational qualities of Rogers' Principles of Homeodynamics and the conceptualisation of invisible and dynamic energy fields continued to be integrated into my thoughts as I entered professional nursing (Fig. 3.1). I retained what I had been taught and was eager to now apply the knowledge to patients as I started my first job as a registered nurse on the gynaecology unit at Memorial Sloan-Kettering Cancer Center in New York City. I was fortunate to have had the choice to work at almost any hospital in the city and select my favourite client group. I was always

Fig. 3.1 Dripstone Crags, Northern Territory photo by Marilynne N. Kirshbaum

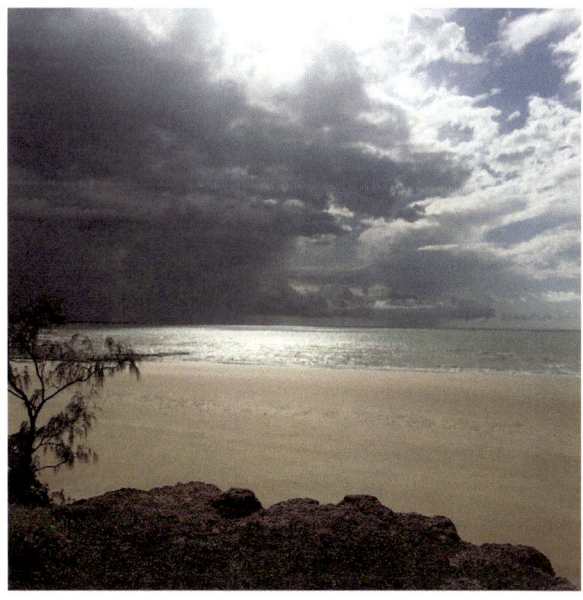

© Springer Nature Switzerland AG 2021
M. N. Kirshbaum, *The Joyful Freedom Approach to Cancer-Related Fatigue*,
https://doi.org/10.1007/978-3-030-76932-1_3

fascinated by people who had neurological conditions because they perceived and experienced their surroundings through sometimes quite bizarre alterations in their senses. The desire was strong to work on a neurological unit, be it medical, surgical or intensive care, where I would have the opportunity to promote well-being of the human energy fields that fascinated me most. However, I decided to accept a job offer in the specialty of oncology nursing, at a top cancer centre, where nursing was renowned for being more advanced, autonomous and specialist. The nurses at Sloan-Kettering pioneered the implementation of nursing, rather than medical diagnosis. Nursing diagnoses were at the core of the nursing care plan, which meant that we planned care around patient problems that could be addressed by nursing interventions. Doctors made their own diagnoses according to the treatments they were qualified to provide. In practice, this meant that a surgeon would mostly focus on the details of their prescribed surgery, whereas as a nurse, I would be focusing on promoting healing of the surgical incision, for example assessing the wound and keeping it clean and infection-free, ensuring the person received adequate hydration and nourishment and promoting comfort in terms of positioning, analgesia and adequate rest. I started off as a Clinical Nurse 1, with a 6-month probation period at Sloan-Kettering. I was ambitious and ready to take on the challenges that awaited me.

3.2   Observation and Actions in Practice

From day one, I was exposed to state-of-the-art cancer treatments, where high doses of toxic chemotherapy and radiotherapy were given, and inconceivable disfiguring surgical procedures were performed on people from all over the world. Often, the patients in my care did not speak much English. However, I felt they were able to see and directly benefit from the compassionate attentiveness that I tried to infuse into my actions throughout every shift. It was tough—of course it was—I was a novice nurse and had a steep learning curve to climb that involved applying the knowledge gained from the university experience to caring for many very ill and emotionally distraught patients and their families.

It is hard to reflect on my early practice with true objectivity; there was quite a bit happening in my life at the same time. My mum had recently died from stomach cancer, a romantic relationship was heating up and I was exposed to the phenomenon known as 'burn out' as I shadowed a more experienced nurse who was suffering in silence, trying to hold it together for the keen 'little nurse' who followed her around asking lots of questions, all day long. I hoped I was not being too annoying, but I was also just 23 years old and knew there was so much that I needed to learn. I was also at a stage where I was driven to pack in as much as I could each and every day while I was still living in New York City. There must have been a hint that I would be moving on.

I would like to spend a bit of time writing about observation as a nurse and researcher, where there is a specific, identified information gathering purpose. In these situations, all our senses can be called upon to assess objectively using measurement tools (e.g. thermometers, sphygmomanometers and validated quality of life questionnaires), subjectively through communication (verbal, non-verbal and touch) and intuitively using our inner guidance.

In nursing practice, observation along with constant ongoing assessment and attentiveness to a client or patient's emotional, mental or physical status is pretty much the cornerstone of care. Along with observation, we can begin to feel and use our intuitive senses to better respond and address a person's needs that might save their life or prevent them from experiencing unnecessary pain and suffering.

Observation, particularly close observation with full attention and intention, is a true privilege. It is an activity that demands to be carried out with utmost respect and honour for those who are at the centre of care. Observation is also a skill that can be practiced and honed with time—if we, as healthcare practitioners and researchers put in the effort and attention.

I have always been a keen observer of the rich diversity of people in New York mostly while walking through different districts and neighbourhoods and riding the subway. My curiosity and creative perceptions led to quite intricate short story writing about some great characters. I had plenty of rich material right in front of me. Sometimes, I managed to do quick portrait drawings, trying to remember to be sensitive to people and not be too obvious. I got caught out a few times and once the other person was sketching me, sketching him—that was interesting!

Observation of an identified phenomenon is the first step in any scientific study. What is that? What does it look like that? Or behave, move or react like that? Then, we decide to take a closer look and observe and record our observations—scientifically. It is assumed that once we analyse our data, the world will be a little more knowledgeable and perhaps wiser. But then we will be drawn to ask more questions to understand the phenomenon a bit better, which will then lead to the generation of further questions, and so it goes.

The same is true for healthcare professionals. I believe that most are pretty keen observers of people in particular, but some might not even realise how integral it is to most of what they do while on the job. I am so grateful though to have been given the opportunity as a student to be removed from the 'doing' part of patient care on the ward and told to just place myself out of way and observe the neonatal intensive care unit (NICU) for a few hours and to take notes of what I saw. I sat in a corner, observed intently and took some notes. I noticed the movements of the nurses, doctors, pharmacists and physios as they looked at charts, made their assessments, talked to each other, used various equipment and interacted with each other and the parents of the tiniest babies that miraculously survived and were being cared for with all the greatest expertise available at a large teaching hospital. I noticed the way hospital personnel played out their designated professional roles through their actions and how much time was spent chatting, trying to find the equipment they needed, looking at their watches and writing in their charts. I remember noticing that some nurses did lots of walking and kept a steady flow of busyness, while others seemed a bit more sedate and moved more slowly but seemed to be much more efficient. There was lots of writing going in charts, on labels and on little slips of paper. I did not know what they were writing or what they were thinking. I stayed in my seat and noticed the flow of activity.

There were times of great hustle and bustle and movement and then times when it was quiet except for the sounds of the ventilators that puffed air in and released air out of tiny lungs, heart monitors that beeped, buzzed and pinged according to their uniquely identifiable sound and frequency. My curiosity was sparked, and I wondered if I would ever be a qualified nurse and have the confidence and skill to do what these nurses in front of me were doing.

I remembered travelling along the path of a nursing student at New York University. Martha Rogers Theory prevailed over the curriculum structure, through all lessons, assignments and exams. I was enthralled and completely fascinated by using the framework to observe, assess and structure the planning of all nursing care for each individual patient [= human energy field]. For example, an older person's extensive wrinkles were not viewed as being degenerative but described in terms of increasing in complexity—and a natural repatterning of the human field as a result of lowered levels of collagen. Practically, the obsession of some traditional, 'old-fashioned' nurses had with tidiness was similarly reframed. For example, it is important to keep a patient's side table clean and clear because that was a way of energising the person's immediate space-time environment. The integration of Rogerian Principles into nursing observations and interventions was reflected in writing extensive and detailed nursing care plans. Therefore, in addition to the standard headings of the nursing process: assessment, problem/nursing diagnosis, action/intervention, outcome and comments, there were columns that corresponded to each principle that had to be completed. So, for example, if the patient had a urinary tract infection, nursing students who were studying at NYU at that time had to consider how to address the problem in terms of *reciprocity* and *synchronicity*, which required quite a bit of creativity and imagination. Well, if *synchronicity* is concerned with relationships in space-time, then I would write something about the relationship between the invading bacteria causing the infection feeding off the person's urine and the plan to introduce targeted antibiotics to kill the harmful bacteria. For a complete entry into the care plan, I would write something about monitoring the effects of the treatment integrating the element of time, for example, the need to record the patient's temperature hourly.

The patients in my care were sentient, complex, multidimensionally, whole beings contained in a permeable unseen yet subtly felt boundary as an energy field. I too existed within an energy field that was unique to me. Our fields would merge during physical care through touch as I would take their blood pressure, help them get comfortable in bed, change their dressings on a wound or drain and also do lots of listening and some talking. I explored and experimented on how I could make their environment as therapeutic and as conducive to healing as possible. It came naturally I suppose, but I would have Rogers' framework buzzing around my brain. I would be taking notes on how I was altering the space-time in the room by tidying the bedside table and decluttering the surrounding area, supporting homeodynamic principles through encouraging the person to drink some more water or offering to bring in some other beverage if that would help. And of course, keep a close eye on intravenous fluids.

Energy fields were also relevant when a psycho-social issue was noticed, and sensitive and genuinely interested listening was required to encourage the expression of worries and fears. At these times, building trust and emitting compassion for another would be required as the energy fields of patient and nurse would meet and interact.

It was all energy then, and it made complete sense to me as I cared for cancer patients from all over the world, many undergoing cutting-edge treatments and many of whom experienced a great deal of suffering. I was still very much a novice nurse then and was driven and encouraged to learn and understand more and more. Although I had learnt plenty about nursing, there was still so much that was unknown. Eventually, I started formulating formal research questions and doing my own empirical research Step by step, I was advancing but without a strategic plan. I was getting experience 'in practice' and adhering to the Principle of Helicy [life as a spiral].

Fast forward now from the super city with its bright lights and diverse, international population to a small semi-rural village in South Yorkshire, England, where I remained for 30 years. I married a man from Manchester (whom I met in New York), completed two higher degrees in nursing, mothered two healthy children and held various posts in nursing and higher education, including a position as a specialist research nurse in breast care and oncology at a local district general hospital. This was a critical turning point for me professionally.

I started as a research nurse working part-time, alongside a Breast Care Specialist Nurse on a newly established 10-bedded breast care unit. Here, I was caring for people, mainly women, who had breast cancer or were at high risk of developing breast cancer, in the context of clinical trials of new chemotherapeutic, hormonal and immunotherapeutic agents. The core part of the position was helping people make the big decision about whether to participate in a clinical trial of a new treatment, which might be more effective or have less side effects than the standard treatment, administer the chemotherapy treatment according to the strictly defined protocol and review the participant's tolerance to the drug, record adverse reactions and quality of life assessments, sometimes take blood samples and provide ongoing supportive, sensitive, empathetic counselling as required. I loved every moment.

3.3   Unearthing Cancer-related Fatigue

From an energetic perspective, the human field of those affected by cancer would be challenged to maintain integrity. As the field is permeable, even visiting a hospital and succumbing to blood tests, X-rays, scans and the disinfected corridors and sterile clinical rooms places demands on the person who is trying to cope with the discomfort, pain and seriousness of every visit. Think of how different you feel when you are in the park or the woods, on the beach, on top of a mountain or in the comfort of your lounge when compared to a hospital clinic or having to hold still and relax as the phlebotomist fills numerous plastic vials with your blood. Can you visualise the quality of the permeable energy field in these situations? In pleasant surroundings, the energy field is soaking up all the nourishment from the air and earth, but in hospital surroundings, there is usually a tightness, a holding or shielding that is functioning to protect us from the discomfort and the unknown of the external clinical environment. Here, healthcare professions can do more than function competently; they can demonstrate compassion and kindness through their actions and words, which can help to put a person at their ease through the emission of soothing and caring vibrations.

I truly loved working as a research nurse and then in the research manager role, in a specialist unit as part of an exceptional multidisciplinary team. It turns out I was very lucky, landing at the right place at the right time. The inspiration from clinical practice for the original research that would lead me to my life's work was revealed. I held onto Rogers' Conceptual Framework and while attending to the women on the Breast Unit and observed the physical and mental consequences associated with living with a diagnosis of cancer I realised that just about everyone experienced a loss or almost total depletion of healthy, vibrant, life-force energy.

A significant part of the research nurse job involved conducting weekly, monthly and yearly assessments of clinical trial participants. I observed and recorded over and over again that there was an almost universal physical, cognitive and emotional problem that was not being heard ardently and certainly not being addressed seriously enough by healthcare professionals. The women in the breast clinic, both those who were participating in clinical trials and those who were not, kept telling me about a vague form of lethargy and tiredness that seemed to prevail in all aspects of their lives. This was being observed all the way from an often traumatic and life-changing diagnosis moment, through their cancer treatment pathway and continued long after treatment had ended. This was a curious observation as although they were considered well and 'disease free' according to their doctors, mammograms, scans and blood tests, there was a continuing and distressing problem that existed under the surface which needed attention.

Anyone who has lived with cancer is familiar with the often overwhelming, frustrating, devastating and multidimensional sensations of fatigue. It is an unwelcomed and frequently unexpected adjunct to the disease that may appear suddenly, without fair warning, when out having fun, enjoying the company of others or participating in a gentle, pleasurable and seemingly undemanding activity. Still, for the person who is trying their utmost to cope with a potentially life-threatening and generally feared aberration of cell proliferation, there will most likely be very little that modern medicine can do to address this kind of fatigue. I remember how upsetting it was for me to witness repeatedly the call for help from cancer patients who reported how helpless they felt as a result of feeling so tired and dysfunctional all the time and then to be told by their doctor that they should feel happy that their mammogram was clear, and they should feel grateful to be alive. The medical response was to rule out anaemia by ordering a blood test and advise their patient to rest and 'put up' with the tiredness.

I continued to ask about the side effects of experimental and standard drug treatment regimens and record their incidences and severity because it was part of my job in clinical research. Troubling fatigue was often mentioned and recorded, but there was not much research evidence around at the time that could inform me on ways to help these women. This was until the ward sister showed me an article about the benefits of exercise for cancer-related fatigue (CRF). Well, that started me on the area of inquiry that I am still following, decades later. I remain in pursuit of knowledge about CRF and have devoted many years researching what can be done to restore energy when it has been depleted by illness. This is also applicable to enlivening those who suffer from lethargy and fatigue following significant life-changing events. The first step for me in practice at this time was to observe how fatigue was experienced and managed within the breast care unit and beyond and then to gather research knowledge about all aspects of CRF.

3.4   What Is Cancer-related Fatigue?

Through observation, reading and smallscale research studies, I found out that cancer-related fatigue (CRF) is so much more than feeling tired or worn down from the stress of living in the modern world. First, it is important to be reminded that fatigue is a subjective experience that varies in intensity from moment to moment in response to shifts in mood, stimulation and hormonal and biochemical regulation. Fatigue is described by people who have cancer as tiredness, weakness, lack of energy, exhaustion, lethargy and depression. Fatigue is the sensation characterised by the lead-weight heaviness felt in one's arms and legs or in the neck as one notices how hard it is to hold one's head up and balance it between the shoulders. Talking becomes an effort as it can become a strain to move the chest and push the air past the vocal cords. There can be a constant battle with one's eyelids to stay open and not succumb or be rude to the person you are with in the middle of a conversation, meal or film. Everything, even the most basic and routine activity, can become such a massive effort, and this can be hugely distressing.

It is human nature to compare the present with the past, when, for example washing the kitchen floor took 10 min and was no big deal—and now it is close to impossible; you need to ask someone to help or put up with a dirty floor. Neither is acceptable, but the person with CRF needs to find ways to change their attitude and behaviours and find a way to avoid or lessen the emergence of a negative self-view, characterised by frustration, helplessness and often low-grade depression.

In the research literature, fatigue is cited as being the most frequently reported symptom of cancer and cancer treatment. It is also the most challenging symptom-management problem for both medical and allied health professionals, which can indirectly impact disease progression. Understanding and treating fatigue is particularly difficult because it is multidimensional: It includes a physical component of decreased functional status, an affective component of emotional distress and a cognitive component that makes concentrating and communicating difficult.

Definitions of CRF abound in the medical and nursing literature. This one from the American National Comprehensive Cancer Network (NCCN) is one of the best, as it is evidenced-based, comprehensive and functional, followed by my own working definition.

Cancer-related fatigue is a distressing, persistent, subjective sense of physical, emotional and/or cognitive tiredness or exhaustion related to cancer or cancer treatment that is not proportional to recent activity and interferes with usual functioning' (NCCN 2019, FT-1)

***

Practically, CRF is distinguished from the more familiar experience of tiredness because it is not relieved easily by addressing a deficiency such as sleep, food or water. It is an individual complex and subjective experience that is prolonged, relentless, at times overwhelming and may vary in intensity and duration (Kirshbaum 2010, p. 214)

Bootsma et al.'s (2019) meta-ethnography presented a welcomed review of studies that provided 'an overarching interpretive narrative on patients' experiences and responses to chronic cancer related fatigue (CCRF)' (p. 1). The authors utilised the term CCRF to focus on the fatigue that persists months and years following treatment. This is the characteristic of fatigue that holds particular interest to me. The authors offered a conceptual view expressed as six meta-themes: *embodied experience, (mis)recognition, small horizon, role change, loss of self* and *regaining one's footing*. The themes were not universal across all individuals; however, conceptually, Bootsma et al.'s (2019) deepened and broadened understanding of the experience in a novel way. The theme *embodied experience* established that the experience of CCRF was mainly to do with bodily sensations or symptoms, for example heavy limbs, wobbly legs or a body that cannot heal nor function well. *(Mis)recognition* concerned the aspect of fatigue, which is not obvious to onlookers, including healthcare professionals. This is associated with the subjective nature of the problem, which can camouflage the struggle due to the lack of objective measures that are more readily addressed by the medical establishment and much of society. *Small horizon* captured the change in perspective and actual functional roles that accompany fatigue. The world of the individual contracts and is diminished as all activities become more difficult and take on the characteristics of obstacles that get in the way of life. *Role change* occurs when the CCRF affects the ability of the person to carry out their usual roles. They become more dependent, more likely to reduce or stop working and become less active socially. The theme of *loss of self* provided awareness for being faced with having to come to terms with illness and physical discomfort. It constitutes a change in identity and behaviour for many. My interpretation of *regaining one's footing* rests in noticing the innate will of the person to return to normal using previous strategies to adapt to disruptive changes, for example fix the problem, distract themselves or conceal the symptom. Here lays one of the gems of this work for me, which aligns with the evolving *Energy Restoration Framework*; there is an innate drive of the person to manage their fatigue in a way that works for them. The key is in helping them to discover an individualised array of approaches and determine when and under which circumstances they are likely to be effective for them. Now that sounds achievable—and it is. But first it is necessary to be aware of the multiple causes behind the multidimensional side effects and symptoms of CRF.

3.5   What Causes Cancer-related Fatigue?

There is only one truly objective measure that validates someone's persistent call for professional advice about how to manage extreme tiredness or fatigue that is not relieved by sleep. This is anaemia, evidenced by a low blood haemoglobin count and treatable by a transfusion of whole blood, blood products or a replenishment of iron. However, there is a multitude of other causes, some of which are not obvious to the person or practitioners that co-exist along the cancer trajectory.

I spent many years working with the charity Breast Cancer Care in the United Kingdom facilitating workshops for women who had breast cancer. I often started the sessions going through the path of cancer diagnosis, treatment and survivorship and exposed the stark reality that just about everything they have been through in the past weeks or months has challenged their natural homeostasis by placing huge demands upon them from all directions. This would have affected their usual ability to collect and utilise the infinite energetic resources normally available in great quantity all around them (see Figs. 3.2 and 3.3).

At every stage of the cancer trajectory, the human energy field gets battered. The deleterious effect increases over time as additional threats to healthy vitality are faced as part of the cancer experience. It is a bit obvious, but to start with, cancer itself exists to draw energy from the physical body. The mutated cell invades a healthy body part, attempts to replicate often at a frenetic speed and causes havoc wherever it is situated. If it invades a solid tumour, the size, weight and biochemical load will steadily increase,

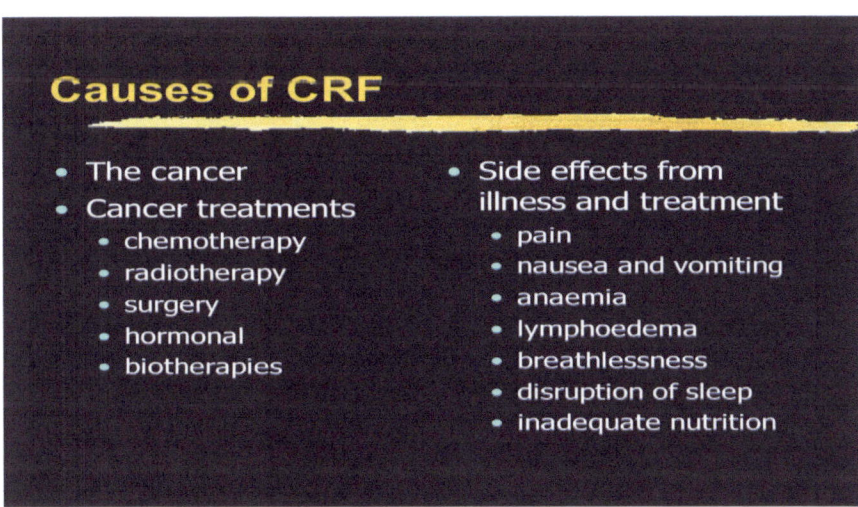

Fig. 3.2 Causes of cancer-related fatigue

EFFECTS OF DIAGNOSIS AND TREATMENT
ALL PATHS (SIDE EFFECTS) LEAD TO FATIGUE

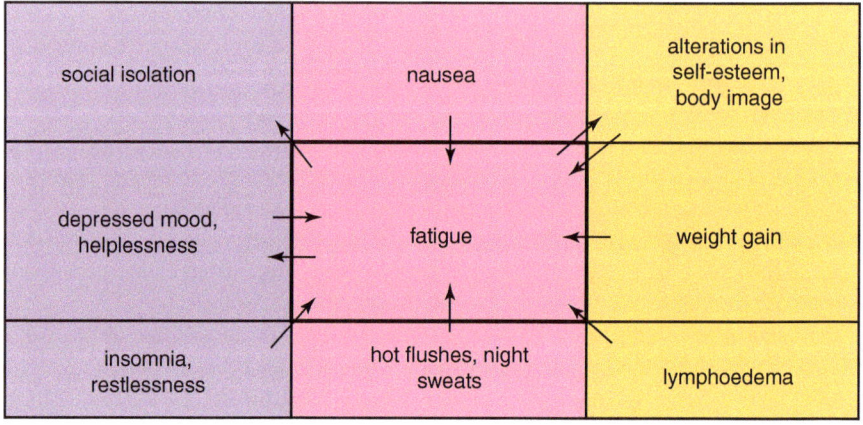

Fig. 3.3 Effects of diagnosis and treatment: all paths (side effects) lead to fatigue

deplete energy reserves and become a noticeable burden physically and also emotionally, as worry, anxiety, fear and depression are initiated by the reality of the active, growing and invading foreign entity. Furthermore, the diagnostic phase is often accompanied by more uncertainty, worry, fear and sometimes annoyance with the bureaucratic inefficiencies of the health service and hospital processes, in addition to the discomfort of diagnostic tests such as mammograms, biopsies, scans and blood tests.

Then, once a definitive diagnosis has been made, there may be an option to enter a clinical trial that may offer an alternative approach or regime to standard treatment. The person will need to listen and try to understand different treatment choices. This takes concentration and depletes mental, cognitive energy and normally is best considered, discussed and decided without too much delay because the cancer cells do not take a 'time out', while the person is weighing up the pros and cons of different treatment options.

Notoriously, the most obvious causes of fatigue and extreme tiredness are the traditional cytotoxic [cancer-cell killing] treatments: chemotherapy and radiotherapy. For some cancers, bone marrow transplantation is the treatment of choice, where extremely high doses of chemotherapy and/or radiation are given followed by the transfusion of precursor blood cells that will replace the almost total amelioration of cancerous and vital blood cells. These therapies are administered to kill cancer cells and in the process also cause much damage to other sensitive cells, such as those lining the digestive track, hair follicles and blood cells. The result for the person is that cancer cells are killed [hopefully], but the corresponding side effects of nausea and vomiting, alopecia, anaemia, neutropenia and immunosuppression are also evident. The anaemia will be expressed as fatigue, reported to a healthcare professional and then an appropriate treatment such as an immediate blood transfusion can be prescribed and swiftly improve the person's wellbeing.

Aside from anaemia, which is detectable through a blood test, the actual pathophysiological mechanisms of CRF are unproven; however, many are proposed and have been investigated. These would include pro-inflammatory cytokines (Collado-Hidalgo et al. 2006; Bower and Lamkin 2013), hypothalamic–pituitary–adrenal axis regulation deregulation (Miller et al. 2008; Bower et al. 2005), circadian rhythm desynchronisation (Berger and Farr 1999), skeletal muscle wasting (Al-Majid and McCarthy 2001) and genetic dysregulation (Rich 2007).

Other cancer treatments such as surgery, hormonal therapy and immune-biological therapies can also contribute to fatigue. Let us focus on surgery. In the cancer world, it can be curative—definitively curative, if the operation to remove the cancerous tumour is done before any metastases have occurred. And that is so wonderful! Yet, the whole process entails energy-zapping events. First, preparing for surgery will usually be stressful. It includes coming to terms with acknowledging that there is a cancer that has invaded the body—this is scary—even if it is the size of a tiny pea. Clearing one's diary of obligations and responsibilities adds more stress to the situation. Then thinking about staying in the hospital may present more worry, for example: Will I catch a methicillin-resistant bug? How will I be able to sleep in a hospital bed and ward? What if the surgeon finds that the tumour has grown larger or has infiltrated a vital organ? Some folks may be very concerned about the anaesthetic and possible nausea afterwards. I remember being quite anxious about this when I had major surgery. It is noteworthy to mention that the anaesthetic is not just one drug, but a cocktail of several different compounds and strong pharmaceuticals that will disrupt the perfect biochemical balance of an otherwise healthy body. There are also prophylactic antibiotics to consider. All of these substances that are infused into the body will affect the integrity of the whole-body system and act to deplete rather than fortify the energy stores of the person.

For those who are treated for breast, ovarian or prostate cancer, hormonal therapies are prescribed to target the production of hormones in an effort to alter the internal environment by making it less hospitable to cancer cells. Although hormonal treatments are not cytotoxic, they do alter the hormonal balance and have their own set of disruptive and annoying side effects that indirectly contribute to fatigue. For example, the reduction of oestrogen will be accompanied by hot flashes and night sweats that disrupt sleep and cognitive concentration and also cause a loss of libido and difficulty or inability to orgasm.

Relatively recently, compared to the highly established treatments mention previously, immuno-biological therapies have entered the scene as an entirely new branch of medical treatment with tremendous beneficial effects and only minimal side effects. The symptoms described are often called 'flu-like symptoms', which compared to the sometimes life-threatening effects of chemotherapy (e.g. cardiotoxicity, severe neutropenia resulting in septicaemia) are minimal. Yet, we are talking about all over achiness, fever and fatigue, which collectively add to more energy depletion.

The next grouping of contributors to energy depletion are the actual side effects of cancer and its treatments. Here, I am talking about the way the physical, mental, emotional, spiritual and sexual aspects of the person react to and attempt to cope with chronic and acute pain, nausea, vomiting, breathlessness, insomnia, lymphoedema, loss of appetite, alteration in taste, malnourishment and deconditioning of muscles—just to name some of the most common ones. There are others, of course depending on the treatment and individual response. Each side effect presents unique challenges and adjustments to lifestyle and previously 'normal' routines. Addressing these challenges on top of everything else requires focused attention, which is energy-depleting.

The psycho-social effects of living with cancer can be devastating, such as helplessness, fear, depression, depressed mood, anxiety, altered body image, altered self-esteem and social isolation. Socio-economic consequences of illness such as loss of a job, changes in employment status or options and loss of income are financial strains that compound worry and negative stress. Some psycho-social and physical side effects feature within recognised cancer symptom clusters, where some investigators have located their research (Valentine and Meyers 2001; Sarenmalm et al. 2014; Fox et al. 2020). This approach provides a real-world approach to identify and attempt to manage several commonly occurring problems together: for example any combination of depression, anxiety, pain, insomnia and fatigue.

Also, worth mentioning here is the relationship between different side effects and symptoms; it is very likely that they will not only be experienced concurrently but affect each other (Fig. 2.3). For example, if someone is suffering with the discomfort and body-image issues of lymphoedema, it is very likely that they will reduce socialising and if this goes on for a while, it is possible that they will lose their friends and social contacts and experience social isolation. Social isolation could then move the person to feel lonely or depressed.

The spiral of low mood, lethargy, pain, discomfort, worry and insomnia can all co-exist and feed upon each other. This is the reality of cancer-related fatigue—it is very real—there are many different causes and often occurs simultaneously as you can see.

References

Al-Majid S, McCarthy DO. Cancer-induced fatigue and skeletal muscle wasting: the role of exercise. Bio Res Nurs. 2001;2:186–97. Available at http://www.ncbi.nih.gov/pubmed/11547540

Berger A, Farr L. The influence of daytime inactivity and nighttime restlessness on cancer-related fatigue. Oncol Nurs Forum. 1999;26:1663–71.

Bootsma T, Schellekens MPJ, Woezik RAM, Lee ML, Slatman J. Experiencing and responding to chronic cancer-related fatigue: a meta-ethnography of qualitative research. Psycho-Oncology. 2019;29(2):241–50. https://doi.org/10.1002/pon.5213.

Bower JE, Lamkin DM. Inflammation and cancer-related fatigue: mechanism, contributing factors and treatment implications. Brain Behav Immunol. 2013;30(suppl):S48–57.

Bower J, Ganz PA, Aziz N. Altered cortisol response to psychologic stress in breast cancer survivors with persistent fatigue. Psychosom Med. 2005;67:277–80.

Collado-Hidalgo A, Bower J, Ganz PA, Cole S, Irwin MR. Inflammatory biomarkers for persistent fatigue in breast cancer survivors. Clin Cancer Res. 2006;12:2759–66.

Fox RS, Ancoli-Israel S, Roesch SC, et al. Sleep disturbance and cancer-related fatigue symptom cluster in breast cancer patients undergoing chemotherapy. Support Care Cancer. 2020;28:845–55. https://doi.org/10.1007/s00520-019-04834-w.

Kirshbaum M. Cancer-related fatigue: a review of nursing interventions. Br J Community Nurs. 2010;15(5):214–9.

Miller AH, Ancoli-Israel S, Bower J, Capuron L, Irwin MR. Neuroendocrine-immune mechanism in behavioral comorbidities in patients with cancer. J Clin Oncol. 2008;26:971–82.

National Comprehensive Cancer Network (NCCN). NCCN guidelines version 2019: cancer-related fatigue; 2019.

Rich TA. Symptom clusters in cancer patients and their relation to EGFR ligand modulation of the circadian axis. J Support Care Oncol. 2007;5:167–74. Available at: http://www.ncbi.nlm.nih.gov/pubmed/17500504.

Sarenmalm EK, Browall M, Gaston-Johansson F. Symptom burden clusters: a challenge for targeted symptom management. A longitudinal study examining symptom burden clusters in breast Cancer. J Pain Symptom Manag. 2014;47(4):731–41. https://doi.org/10.1016/j.jpainsymman.2013.05.012.

4.1   Introduction

It feels like I have been questing for ways to help people feel well and live their life to their truest and most invigorated potential for most of my adult life, and you know what, I have. The topic continues to intrigue me as I pursue the area with strength and determination (Fig. 4.1). It fills me with delight to observe a steady stream of research articles that have pursued and contributed to this shared goal to not only improve 'well-being', such a generalised term, but have deliberately delved in creatively to address cancer-related fatigue from different vantages and experimental approaches. There is still much research that needs to be done to channel accessible and infinite 'life-force'

Fig. 4.1 The Jaguar by
Carey Vail

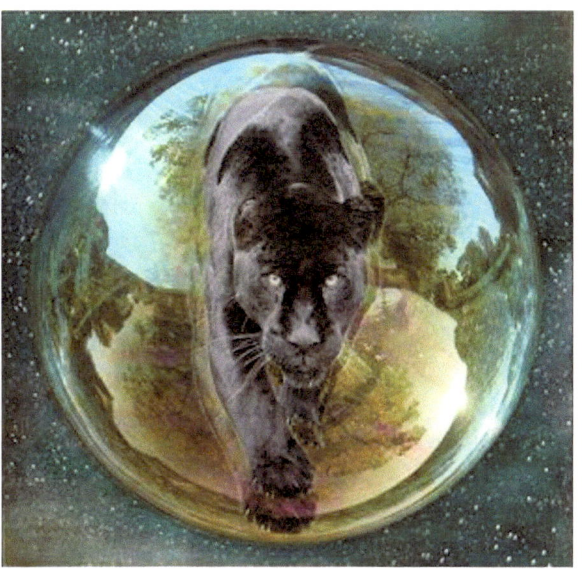

energy into mainstream cancer care. I hope to continue to participate and contribute to extending knowledge and its practical application in the coming years. But, for the time being, I will do my best to systematically review and synthesise what is currently known about how to best approach the multidimensional challenges of cancer-related fatigue.

4.2   Screening and Measurement for Cancer-Related Fatigue

It is so pleasing to see that prominent cancer-care guidelines (Howell et al. 2013, NCCN 2020) are now including baseline screening for fatigue for all cancer patients from the start of cancer treatment and at regular intervals at follow-up clinic visits. This way, the common and expected side effect of all cancers, and most treatments can be monitored effectively, taken seriously and begin to be managed following best-practice guidelines by healthcare professionals. As a screening and monitoring initiative, it is recommended that 'all screening of adults with cancer be conducted using brief, quantitative, self-reported measures with empirically established cut off scores' (Berger et al. 2015, p. 9). Recommended measures are the Edmonton Symptom Assessment System (ESAS) (Bruera et al. 1991) level of tiredness item, where respondents rate their current tiredness on a 1–10 scale or a slightly different single item scale that asks respondents to rate their level of fatigue over the past week. Both approaches conform to using 0 = no tiredness, 1–3 (mild), 4–6 (moderate) and 7–10 (severe) as a guide. When used as a screening tool, the cut-off of 4 is generally accepted as being an indicator of fatigue, which could benefit from intervention and treatment using specific care pathways.

Measurement and full-scale clinical evaluation of fatigue during active treatment and beyond have traditionally been conducted using Quality of Life scales that accompany clinical trials and in other types of clinical oncology research (Yellens et al. 1997; Abrahams et al. 2017). There is therefore much written about a large range of self-reported, subjective scales. Berger et al. (2015) and the NCCN guidelines (2020) provide useful tables that detail the qualities of the measurement tools according to the number of items, validation and specific outcomes (e.g. physical and mental fatigue, motivation and sleep/rest).

4.3   Medical and Pharmacological Treatments

I mentioned previously that if anaemia was found to be the culprit behind continued complaints of persistent low energy and feeling awful so much of the time without relief, then a straightforward medical solution would be to replace the iron and/or precursor in the biochemical/hormonal process by a transfusion of whole blood or an erythropoiesis-stimulating agent and growth factor such as epoetin. Epoetin, a synthetic erythropoietin, is a hormonal growth factor that can be administered routinely as a prophylactic infusion alongside high-dose chemotherapy when severe neutropenia is expected. It has also been used and confirmed by research to increase vigour in severe anaemia (Djubegovic 2005). However, please note that patients will need to be informed of the increased risk of developing thromboembolism (Rizzo et al. 2010); physiological monitoring is advised here.

Other medical or pharmaceutical agents are sometimes prescribed although they have only slight beneficial effects for a minority of recipients along with several established side effects—these are usually best avoided. I wrote a critical summary of a Cochrane Review entitled Pharmacological Treatments for Fatigue Associated with Palliative Care (Kirshbaum 2011). The review looked at medical stimulants and found the psychostimulant modafinil was only slightly helpful and was associated with mild side effects of nausea and vomiting. This was refuted by others (Spathis et al. 2014 and Hovey et al. 2014) who both concluded that there was no benefit in the context of CRF. Another drug in the same category called armodafinil was tolerated better and reduced fatigue for those who had radiotherapy, although the results were not statistically significant (Page et al. 2015). According to yet another source (Gong et al. 2014), methylphenidate was found to have some effect on wakefulness, alongside reports of anxiety, poor sleep and decreased appetite. Hence, there is a balancing act to consider under this approach and a careful decision made under the guise of a prescribing medical or specialist nurse practitioner. The conclusion at this point is that in addition to psychostimulants, there are other treatments and interventions to examine that will most probably be more suitable for longer term use and for overall improvement in general well-being and health.

The next group of pharmacologic approaches, are the powerful, affordable and wondrously versatile glucocorticoids, commonly known as steroids such as prednisolone and dexamethasone. These too have been prescribed and investigated for their potential benefit for CRF (Minton et al. 2010; Kirshbaum 2011; Mücke et al. 2015) in addition to their known efficacy in stimulating appetite, wound healing, reducing nausea and pain relief. Both dexamethasone and methylprednisolone can provide some relief in the short term, particularly when multiple problems and side effects of cancer are evident or indeed COVID19. [Dexamethasone has been a game-changer in 2020, attributed with reducing the severity and advancement of the virus during the pandemic that started in 2020]. But remember long-term use of steroids is dangerous and not advisable because of their undesirable effects on sleep, weight gain due to increased appetite (with a preference for high-calorific sweet and fatty foods), association with depression and serious muscle wasting with progressive use (Yennurajalingam et al. 2013; Yennurajalingam and Bruera 2014).

Other groups of medicines such as antidepressants, specifically selective serotonin reuptake inhibitors (SSRIs) such as fluoxetine (Prozac), paroxetine (Paxil, Pexeva) and sertraline (Zoloft), and cholinesterase inhibitors like donepezil (Aricept; commonly used by people who are living with Alzheimer's Disease), might still be found to be effective by tackling fatigue through a lateral or comorbidity pathway, such as depression. However, for the moment, I suggest we turn our attention to the vast expanse of non-medical approaches. This is where it gets interesting for me as there are so many possibilities and combinations of modalities that can be explored, tested and used to assist people to regain some of the control over their own bodies, lost within the medical–surgical approach to diagnosis and primary treatments. I hope your curiosity is kindled sufficiently to read on …

4.4   Non-Medical Approaches and Interventions

As a nurse with a leaning toward non-medicalised and holistic health practice, my interest was and still is in discovering and exploring the seemingly infinite possibilities of interventions that can be facilitated by healthcare practitioners to address all levels of cancer-related fatigue. In my article, *Cancer-related fatigue: A review of nursing interventions* (Kirshbaum 2010), I identified 436 titles of research articles that appeared to be relevant to the search question: 'Which strategies and interventions aimed at the management of cancer-related fatigue should be promoted by community practitioners?' After a critical quality review and selection, only 61 empirical studies and 4 systematic reviews (Stone 2002; Mitchell et al. 2007; Cramp and Daniel 2008; Radbrusch et al. 2008) were included in the systematic review at the time. Box 4.1 presents examples of the wide range of approaches evaluated in these research studies. I have also included additional interventions that I have come across while reviewing new research and guidelines.

These varied types of interventions and approaches are grouped into five categories identified as physical activity, adjustment strategies, complementary therapies and psycho-social educational interventions. The same five categories of interventions remain more or less representative regarding this most current and necessary updated review of recent studies, reviews and guidelines. It is exciting and energising for me to discover that the supportive evidence for non-medical interventions is now pleasingly more rigorous and convincing. However, it must still be noted that just about every article and guideline concludes with a statement that more research is required to substantiate unequivocal recommendations. We must still proceed carefully when providing advice to patients and clients.

Box 4.1 Non-Pharmacological Approaches Considered in the Management of Cancer-Related Fatigue
- *Physical activity*
- *Physical exercise (substantial supportive evidence)*
- *Yoga (substantial supportive evidence)*
- *Qigong**
- *Adjustment (self-management) strategies*
- *Nutrition and hydration*
- *Promotion of quality sleep and rest*
- *Energy conservation*
- *Attention restoration activities*
- *Stress management*
- *Mindfulness-based stress reduction* (substantial supportive evidence)*
- *Relaxation*
- *Diary writing/journaling*
- *Complementary therapies*
  - *Acupuncture and acupressure*
- *Massage (substantial supportive evidence)*

- *Aromatherapy*
- *Bright white light therapy (BWLT)* (possibly)*
- *Psychosocial-educational interventions*
- *Anticipatory guidance and information (substantial supportive evidence)*
- *Cognitive behaviour therapy* (substantial supportive evidence)*
- *Supportive expressive therapies*
- *Nutrition consultation**
  *additions

4.5   Systematic Reviews and Guidelines

I will attempt to synthesise the research evidence behind the most promising interventions as this chapter continues. The research literature surrounding cancer-related fatigue abounds with reports of studies at all levels of reliability, for example case studies, single cohort studies, RCTs and meta-analyses. From the current guidelines and systematic reviews, I have drawn most heavily upon the National Comprehensive Cancer Network (NCCN, 2019, 2020) and Berger et al. (2015) due to their inclusive and thorough approach. The NCCN is a very readable and authoritative publication. I would encourage interested readers and practitioners to go directly to this source for further reference and annual updates, which are so critical in this dynamic area. These guidelines, first published in 2000, emerged from a hugely authoritative multidisciplinary panel of experts, mainly based in the United States. The guidelines consist of extensive research-based discussions and appendices that critique and integrate the best evidence for practice.

In the most recent offering in the form of an algorithm for care, all cancer patients should receive screening for fatigue, education about its natural history, counselling about general strategies and coached according to a growing number of non-pharmacological interventions that may help during and after cancer treatment. I was so pleased to see the presence of quite a few complementary and psycho-social therapies that were scrutinized for effectiveness based on single empirical studies and systematic reviews/meta-analyses.

Another highly credible resource for treatment guidance is the Cochrane Database of Systematic Reviews [Cochranelibrary.com]. As of the April 2021 newsletter, there were four systematic reviews that are particularly relevant to CRF. If you go to the website, you will probably find other reviews that are of interest and clinically pertinent to you. In the meantime, I would like to draw your attention to these five reviews, where you will find the critiqued research evidence and associated recommendations on these relevant topics.

- Exercise for the management of cancer-related fatigue in adults. Fiona Cramp, James Byron-Daniels. 14 November 2012 (Kirshbaum 2013).
- Psychosocial interventions for reducing fatigue during cancer treatement in adults (Goedendorp et al. 2009). Drug therapy for the management of

cancer-related fatigue. Ollie Minton, Alison Richardson, Michael Sharpe, Matthew Hotopf, Patrick Stone. 7 July 2010

- Educational interventions for the management of cancer-related fatigue in adults. Sally Bennett, Amanda Pigott, Elaine M Beller, Terry Haines, Pamela Meredith, Christie Delaney. 24 November 2016 (Bennett et al. 2016).
- Pharmacological treatments for fatigue associated with palliative care. Martin Mücke, Mochamat Mochamat, Henning Cuhls, Vera Peuckmann-Post, Ollie Minton, Patrick Stone, Lukas Radbruch. 30 May 2015.

So, now you have some references to view, but what are the best ways to address fatigue? I will be following the terminology used in Box 4.1 and add new information from guidelines, reviews and recent literature searches.

4.5.1 Physical Aerobic Activity

By far, still, the most studied and robust evidence supports continuous moderate aerobic exercise defined as increasing the resting heart rate to 50–90%. This can be achieved by running, brisk walking, swimming or cycling. (See Box 4.2 for key points). While I was a research nurse on the breast care unit at the district general hospital in Huddersfield, England, the studious ward sister Rosie, handed me an article purporting the benefits of stationary cycling during the period of active chemotherapy treatment (Winningham 1983). The most noteworthy benefit, which to be honest sounded pretty outrageous at the time, was reduced nausea. This benefit was recognized after just 10 min of stationary cycling. Winningham and her colleagues (Winningham and MacVicar 1988, Mock et al. 1994) were pioneers in this area. Their studies were replicated and joined by a small cadre of nurse researchers whom I followed through my association with the American-based Oncology Nursing Society for many years, all advancing evidence in relation to the benefits and also limitations of physical exercise for people who had cancer. The sample sizes and rigour of the research studies were very small from their inception but have steadily increased over the years, thus becoming more robust and credible.

When I felt ready to take on the challenges of a PhD, I knew I wanted to contribute to the work of these nurse scientists, not only because it was a bit cutting-edge but also because of my lifelong enthusiastic practices of running, walking, cycling, swimming and yoga. The start of a PhD is often a saga, I will spare you that narrative. Let me just say that after several permeations of research proposals through almost a year of intensive discussions with my PhD supervisors, we reached a reasonable consensus. It was quite a tough endeavour—I had to convince my supervisors of a few anecdotal benefits that did not have strong scientific support. There were times when they did not accept the conclusion of published articles because the journal did not have a high enough impact factor or was not known to them. I was laughed at when I postulated that it is likely that there is a connection between body fat and a woman's risk of developing breast cancer; at the time it was postulated, not proven that oestrogen was probably a contributing factor. However, I survived—we got there, eventually … it was agreed finally that I would prepare for an

RCT on how to best educate and influence breast care nurses and specialists to promote exercise to women in their care (Kirshbaum 2004a, b). The title of my thesis from the University of Manchester, UK was: *Disseminating Research Evidence to Breast Care Nurses: The Case of Exercise for Breast Cancer Patients.* The study was in three phases: a national survey of breast care nurses in the United Kingdom on evidence-based practice (Kirshbaum et al. 2004), a conceptual framework based on behaviour change theories (Kirshbaum 2005a) and finally an RCT (Kirshbaum 2008). The intervention was an evidenced-based booklet, *Exercise and Breast Cancer: A Booklet for Breast Care Nurses,* based on a systematic review of the benefits (Kirshbaum 2005b, Kirshbaum 2007). The booklet was targeted to specialist breast care nurses in the United Kingdom in terms of tone and level of the writing, content and perspective. Barriers to exercise such as economic constraints, absence of an exercise partner, lack of transport, lack of childcare and lack of safe surroundings were not only listed but addressed with common-sense suggestions. For example, attending a gym is not accessible or affordable to everyone, running in the dark (early in the morning or from late afternoon in England) is not an option in 'rough areas'—so alternatives needed to be presented. Please seek out the thesis for the full details (Kirshbaum 2004b).

Box 4.2 Key Points from NCCN Guideline for Active Treatment (NCCN 2020, FT-6)

1. *Maintain optimal level of activity*
2. *Cautions in determining level of activity:*
   (a) *Bone metastasis*
   (b) *Thrombocytopenia*
   (c) *Anaemia*
   (d) *Fever, active infection or post-surgery*
   (e) *Late effects of treatment (e.g. cardiomyopathy)*
   (f) *Limitations secondary to metastasis or other comorbid illnesses*
   (g) *Safety issues (assessment of risk or falls)*
3. *Consider initiation and/or encourage maintenance of a physical activity/ exercise program as appropriate per health care provider consisting of cardiovascular endurance (walking, jogging or swimming) and resistance (weights) training.*
4. *Consider referral to rehabilitation: physical therapy, occupational therapy and physical medicine.*
5. *Yoga*

The early evaluative research of physical activity in CRF was almost exclusively single cohort studies in populations of women who had breast cancer during and after cancer treatment, but the enthusiasm and eagerness to progress the research increased its power of evidence was palpable in these foundational articles (e.g. Winningham 1983; Winningham and MacVicar 1988; Stricker et al. 2004). The body of evidence has now extended considerably to include participants who have been diagnosed with colorectal, prostate, lymphoma and hematologic malignancies, undergoing radiotherapy and post stem cell transplant. In addition, the findings of the studies are much more robust and based on larger samples, comparative studies and well-designed RCTs (Kelley and Kelley 2017a, 2017b; NCCN 2020).

To date, the most recent meta-analyses and systematic reviews remain cautious about putting forward detailed recommendations about which exercise is best and under which circumstances (Kelley and Kelley 2017a, 2017b). There is the obvious limitation of prescribing rigid protocols for populations of cancer patients and survivors who differ in terms of the type of cancer, stage of cancer, phase of treatment, comorbidity and, lest we forget, the unique characteristics and preferences of every individual on this planet. However, it is quite clear that regular (at least 30 min several times a week; total of 3–5 hours a week) aerobic, cardiovascular exercise is best performed at a moderate level that produces a safe, tolerable increase in heart rate depending on the level of fitness. The type of activity is best determined according to individual preference. Consistent encouragement and support by healthcare professionals, in addition to family, friends and peers within cancer support groups, can be extremely advantageous, particularly if it is structured, facilitated and shared within a group (Baumann et al. 2017; Leach et al. 2019).

4.5.2 Yoga and Qigong

Both Yoga and Qigong are holistic practices that involve not just movement but also breathing techniques, meditations, dietary aspects and spiritual lifestyle components. Yoga comprises many different forms, which are distinguished by the emphasis placed on muscle and bone alignments, chakras and energy centres, positioning and flow, just to name a few. Similar to physical exercise, there are quite significant variations that could possibly influence outcome measures, although in the CRF literature these differences are often not apparent—the singular word Yoga refers to the entire grouping. Qigong is the energy building and distributing practice associated with Taichi, which is an ancient martial art that also has health benefits. Its effect on fatigue may be indirect, in terms of reducing stress, improving sleep and general well-being.

A fairly recent Cochrane Review (Cramer et al. 2017) concluded that yoga compared to no therapy improved health-related quality of life, reduced fatigue and improved sleep. It was not as effective generally as physical exercise [mainly aerobic] but enough to support practice for people who have cancer and those who cannot participate in aerobic forms of exercise. There is an increasing amount of studies in this area, and the evidence is becoming stronger but still falls short of strong support in most guidelines and protocols. However, it is always important to remember that fatigue, as a cancer side-effect, rarely exists independently. Yoga has been found to reduce depression and fatigue as well, which are important bonuses to consider when purporting supportive interventions. It seems that in women who have breast cancer, at least two yoga sessions a week is enough to record benefits of sleep quality and fatigue (Taso et al. 2014). Other studies focus on the benefits of yogic breathing for cancer-associated symptoms and quality of life (Dhruva et al. 2012) and psychological symptoms such as depression and anxiety (Lanctôt et al. 2016). The NCCN Guideline panel (2020) concluded that yoga is an effective practice for patients who are on active cancer treatment and that evidence based on men and cancers aside from breast cancer is required to fully and conclusively support recommending yoga to a wider population.

4.5.3 Physically Based Therapies

The group of potentially supportive interventions for CRF referred to as *physically based therapies* are those where a practitioner, such as a massage therapist or acupuncturist, performs a treatment on a largely passive receiver. The research supports massage for patients on active treatment and appears to hold great potential for acupressure and acupuncture in terms of reducing CRF (Balk et al. 2009, Molassiotis et al. 2007, Mao et al. 2009), although more conclusive evidence is currently required. Presently, I am involved in two studies based in China, but led from Australia, which will be contributing to this gap in knowledge from the perspective of cancer symptom clusters (Tan et al. 2018).

There are also other interventions that appear in the research literature such as infrared laser moxibustion (ILM) that uses the shrubby herb known as Artemisia vulgaris (moxa) on the acupuncture site. A small but promising RCT showed statistically significant results for fatigue reduction when compared to a sham [fake] intervention that emulated ILM (Mao et al. 2016). Similarly, transcutaneous electrical acupoint stimulation in non-small cell lung cancer patients was also found to reduce fatigue within a small RCT (Hou et al. 2017).

Aromatherapy and Bright White Light Therapy are included in the guidelines, but the evidence of their direct effectiveness remains quite weak. As with other interventions, comfort and stress reduction can be beneficial—it all depends on how the person perceives their potential soothing effects.

4.5.4 Psychosocial–Educational Interventions

The field of possible interventions in addition to exercise and physical therapies widens next as we move on to addressing the multidimensional condition of CRF from an emotional, cognitive and psychological sphere. The most prominent interventions under this heading are anticipatory guidance and information (substantial supportive evidence), Cognitive Behaviour Therapy (substantial supportive evidence) and supportive expressive therapies.

The power of the mind should never be undervalued. Pure science has demonstrated consistently that the mind and body work together continually and constantly through intricate feedback mechanisms to affect all matter of changes within our amazing bodies. The stress response is a well-established example of how the perception of fear stimulates the adrenal gland to increase the production of epinephrine (adrenaline). On the opposing axis of control, deep relaxation and meditative states encourage the body to release norepinephrine which opens up blood vessels throughout the body and allows nutrients to circulate freely to extremities and other non-vital parts.

Other examples are provided by Dr. Bruce Lipton across several books (Lipton and Bhaerman 2009; Lipton 2015) and many papers and video sessions that are readily available online. His visionary and ground-breaking discoveries go way beyond the fight or flight response and are scientifically credible to a certain extent. They are currently not considered conventional or taught in all medical schools. Convincing the mainstream medical establishments to change traditional practices is notoriously slow but not impossible. Lipman's revolutionary experiments, which took place while he was a Professor of Genetics in medical schools are quite mind-blowing. He demonstrated and has eloquently been explaining for over 20 years that the 'mind-body connection' is very real as is the evidence behind epigenetics—they both involve the intricate biological mechanism of highly 'intelligent' and responsive human cells.

Lipton explains that we can modify much of our destiny; our lives are not exclusively determined by genetics at all. Stress management and taking on a way of life that encourages abundance and growth, rather than stagnation, frustration, worry and fear is one of the most critical points.

We will, I believe, come together in a global community. The members of that enlightened community will recognise that we are made in the image of our environment, i.e. that we are divine, and that we have to operate, not in a survival of the fittest manner, but in a way that supports everyone and everything on this planet' (Lipton 2015, p. 217)

Those who have spiritual beliefs often demonstrate higher levels of mental health that are correlated with lower levels of adrenal stress hormones such as cortisol and epinephrine. The miraculous observation here, which was analysed rigorously and statistically, is that there was less suppression of the immune system, which is the key to ongoing health at all levels. This adds to the developing self-care and holistic well-being paradigm that we need to strive towards supporting and working alongside our protective, complex and powerful immune system and to keep ourselves wide open to new ways of how we can do that. New ways to calm our nervous systems will continue to emerge and infiltrate our consciousness and our very real earthy communities (e.g. Poly Vagal Theory). Our physical bodies are designed to regulate themselves. Do you remember learning about homeostasis? For example, the wondrous ability of the human body to maintain our internal temperature within a very small range (36.5–37 degrees) and the automatic processes involved in sweating, breathing, digesting and sexual arousal. We can attempt to control some of these behaviours and responses to stimuli. But if we loosen our control on the subconscious and promote and work with rather than block the body's 'will to survive', we will experience less detrimental emotions. This all comes down to the regulation of the stress hormones. There are so many techniques and methods out there to explore and research. Spiritual belief is a mighty force that can transform chronic feelings of dread, apprehension, helplessness and lack of purpose into a lighter and easier platform from which to lift off and live life fully and joyously!

The examination of interventions that fall into the psycho-social educational is not straightforward. They are varied and have different foci, despite integrating associated concepts. This is from my analytical and theoretically driven mind but also reflected in the reports of meta-analyses, where categorisation adds to the usual challenges of heterogeneity. This is because single studies often use different measurement instruments and questionnaires, samples, sample sizes, settings and variables that affect comparisons and pooling of data.

The most widely evaluated and substantiated approach under this heading is Cognitive Behaviour Therapy (CBT), followed by a very mixed grouping of interventions referred to as Anticipatory guidance and information (Box 4.1). CBT is a cognitive approach to misguided thinking where the client and therapist join forces to uncover the triggers to a negative emotion, such as distress, guilt or sadness on the basis of an unwelcomed behaviour—and then describe the response, which is usually alerting the person to the problem. The therapist and client together are engaged in and explore how to move forward. Its foundation is helping the person to distinguish between an automatic thought and an emotion using a structured and interactive approach. The objective is to identify the trigger and work in steps to transform the unwanted response to more acceptable alternative behaviours (Beck 2011, Westbrook et al. 2011).

An evolution of CBT has occurred since Aaron Beck first presented his alternative treatment paradigm to analytical psychotherapy for anxiety and depression. The highly adaptable model has been used to help those with physical ailments and health deficiencies, including side effects of fatigue from radiotherapy, as Montgomery et al. (2009) report.

CBT skills including how to recognize negative beliefs regarding radiotherapy and/or fatigue (e.g., catastrophizing); the emotional, behavioural, and physical consequences of those beliefs; how to debate such beliefs and change them to more helpful alternatives (Ellis 1994); and how to practice behavioural strategies to manage treatment-related fatigue (including activity scheduling and exercise, as exercise has been demonstrated to be effective in reducing cancer-related fatigue (Kangas et al. 2008). Following this CBT session, participants were given a CBT workbook to review. They were also taught to complete a thought record worksheet (which typically takes less than five minutes to complete) and were asked to complete two of these worksheets per week (during the six-week course of their radiotherapy). The therapist then met with each patient twice per week (for a total of 12 sessions) in the radiation oncology clinic to go over these worksheets (5- to 15-minute sessions). Attendance was perfect, as participants were necessarily present in the radiation oncology clinic to receive their radiotherapy. (Montgomery et al. 2009, p. 320)

4.5.5 Adjustment (Self-Management) Strategies

4.5.5.1 Supportive Expressive Therapies

There is tremendous scope for advancing the integration of activities that are designed to draw out the repressed emotions that most people with cancer hold tight within themselves but in a gentle, supported and expansive way. Much research has documented depression and anxiety independently and within quality-of-life assessments. This is not surprising when we consider that it is normal to experience grief for the loss of health, fear of treatment side-effects or death, anger at anyone who comes close and also periods of self-loathing when looking in the mirror of a surgical scar, the extra body fat that has accumulated, alopecia or sometimes shame for previous bad habits that might have precipitated cancer. From an energic perspective, I will add that it is energy depleting and chronically harmful to pretend that you are well and happy when you are clearly NOT. You will be deceiving yourself and this will stand in the way of moving forward with beneficial action. However, clearing old habits requires commitment to some kind of approach or plan that is acceptable to you. Participation in the visual or performing arts, writing prose or poetry and supportive group sessions lead by skilled fascilitators for the purpose of contained and safe expression of deep emotions have been evaluated with very promising findings (Ennis et al. 2019; Bosman et al. 2020).

These forms of intervention are particularly interesting to me, as I develop a novel program for all forms of energy depletion based on individual responsibility and enjoyment. I am pleased to have identified quite a few programs in the acute and community setting where ongoing programs have been established. These programs have exposed the multidimensional benefits of joy, expansion through learning, sharing and connecting with others and the delight of taking pride in a finished product of beauty (e.g. painting, sculpture, dance and poetry) and through stress management modalities such as mindfulness, meditation and hypnotherapy.

4.5.5.2 Supportive Educational Programs

This approach is often led by healthcare professionals who recognise the importance of health promotion following a cancer diagnosis (e.g. Breast Cancer Care, NT Cancer Council and Singapore Cancer Council). There is plenty of scope for providing an educational program on cancer, side effects of treatment, nutritional advice, sleep hygiene and exercise guidelines. Often integrative therapies such as aromatherapy, reflexology, Qigong, forest bathing or reiki are offered. This approach provides scope for individuals to interact and participate in a structured activity or information exchange. This will have an indirect effect on fatigue by reducing stress, adding an element of distraction but also enjoyment, comfort, social connection and welcomed mental stimulation.

References

Abrahams HJG, Gielissen MFM, De Lugt M, Kleijer EFW, De Roos WK, Balk E, Verhagen, CAHHVM, Knoop H. "The Distress Thermometer for Screening for Severe Fatigue in Newly Diagnosed Breast and Colorectal Cancer Patients". Psycho-oncology (Chichester, England) 26.5. 2017;693–97. Web.

Balk J, Day R, Rosenzweig M, Beriwal S. Pilot, randomized, modified, double-blind, placebo-controlled trial of acupuncture for cancer-related fatigue. J Soc Integr Oncol. 2009 Winter;7(1):4–11.

Baumann FT, Bieck O, Oberest M, et al. Sustainable impact of an individualised exercise program on physical activity level and fatigue syndrome on breast cancer patients in two German rehabilitation centers. Supportive Care in Cancer. 2017;25:1047–54.

Beck JS. Cognitive behaviour therapy: basics and beyond. 2nd ed. New York: Guildford Press; 2011.

Bennett S, Pigott A, Beller EM, Haines T, Meredith P, Delaney C. Educational interventions for the management of cancer-related fatigue in adults. Cochrane Review Library. 2016.

Berger AM, Mitchell SA, Jacobson PB, Pirl WF. Screening, evaluation and management of cancer related fatigue: ready for implementation to practice? Cancer J Clin. 2015;65(3) 10.3322. caac.21268.

Bosman JT, Bood ZM, Scherer-Rath M, et al. The effects of art therapy on anxiety, depression, and quality of life in adults with cancer: a systematic literature review. Support Care Cancer. 2020).; (Art therapy).; https://doi.org/10.1007/s00520-020-05869-0.

Bruera E, Kuehn N, Miller MJ, Selmser P, Macmillan K. The Edmonton symptom assessment system (ESAS): a simple method for the assessment of palliative care patients. J Palliat Care. 1991;7:6–9.

Cramer H, Lauche R, Klose P, Lange S, Langhorst J, Dobos GJ. Yoga for improving health-related quality of life, mental health and cancer-related symptoms in women diagnosed with breast cancer. Cochrane Database Syst Rev. 2017;1(1):CD010802. https://doi.org/10.1002/14651858. CD010802.pub2.

Cramp F, Daniel J. Exercise for the management of cancer-related fatigue in adults. Cochrane Database Syst Rev. 2008;(2):CD006145. https://doi.org/10.1002/14651858.CD006145.pub2.

Dhruva A, Miaskowski C, Abrams D, Acree M, Cooper B, Goodman S, Hecht FM. Yoga breathing for cancer chemotherapy-associated symptoms and quality of life: results of a pilot randomized controlled trial. J Altern Complement Med. 2012;18(5):473–9. https://doi.org/10.1089/acm.2011.0555.

Djubegovic B. Erthythropoeitin use in oncology: A summary of the evidence and practice guidelines comparing efforts of the Cochrane Review group and Blue Cross/Blue Shield to set up the ASCO/Ash guidelines. Best Practice and Research. Clinical Hematology. 2005;18:455-466. as cited by: Mitchell SA, Bock SL, Hood LE, Moore K & Tanner ER. Putting Evidence into Practice: Evidence Based Interventions for Fatigue During and Following Cancer and Its Treatment Clinical Journal of Oncology. 2007;11(1):99–113.

Ellis, A. Reason and emotion in psychotherapy. Secaucus, NJ: Birch Lane. 1994.

Ennis G, Kirshbaum M, Waheed N. The energy-enhancing potential of participatory performance-based arts activities in the care of people with a diagnosis of cancer: an integrative review. Arts Health. 2019;11(2):87–103. https://doi.org/10.1080/17533015.2018.1443951.

Goedendorp MM, Gielissen MF, Verhagen CA, Bleijenberg G. Psychosocial interventions for reducing fatigue during cancer treatment in adults. Cochrane Database Systematic Reviews. 2009:CD06953.

Gong S, Jin S, et al. Effect of methylphenidate in patients with cancer-related fatigue: a systematic review and meta-analysis. PLoS One. 2014;9:e84391.

Hou L, Zhou C, Wu Y, Yu Y, Hu Y. Transcutaneous electrical acupoint stimulation (TEAS) relieved cancer-related fatigue in non-small cell lung cancer (NSCLC) patients after chemotherapy. J Thorac Dis. 2017;9(7):1959–66. https://doi.org/10.21037/jtd.2017.06.05.

Hovey E, de Souza P, Marx G, et al. Phase III, randomized, double-blind, placebo-controlled study of modafinil for fatigue in patients treated with docetaxel-based chemotherapy. Support Care Cancer. 2014;22:1233–42. https://link.springer.com/article/10.1007%2Fs00520-020-05869-0

Howell D, Keller-Olaman S, Oliver TK, et al. A pan-Canadian practice guidelines and algorithm: screening, assessment and supportive care of adults with cancer-related fatigue. Curr Oncol. 2013;20:e233–46.

Kangas M, Bovbjerg DH, Montgomery GH. Cancer-related fatigue: A systematic and meta-analytic review of non-pharmacological therapies for cancer patients. Psychological Bulletin. 2008;34:700–741.

Kelley GA, Kelley KS. Aerobic exercise and cancer-related fatigue in adults: a reexamination using the IVhet model for meta-analysis. Cancer Epidemiol Biomarkers Prev. 2017a;26(2):281–3. https://doi.org/10.1158/1055-9965.EPI-16-0885.

Kelley GA, Kelley KS. Exercise and cancer-related fatigue in adults: a systematic review of previous systematic reviews with meta-analyses. BMC Cancer. 2017b;17(1):693. https://doi.org/10.1186/s12885-017-3687-5.

Kirshbaum M, Beaver K, Luker K. Perspectives of breast care nurses on research dissemination and utilisation. Clin Eff Nurs. 2004;8(1):47–58.

Kirshbaum M, Donbavand J. Making the most out of life: Exploring the contribution of Attention Restorative Theory in developing a non-pharmacological intervention for fatigue. Palliative and Supportive Care 2013;12(6):473–80.

Kirshbaum M. A conceptual framework for targeting research dissemination interventions to meet the needs of breast cancer patients in the United Kingdom. (Published conference abstract). Oncol Nurs Forum. 2005a;32(1):164.

Kirshbaum M. A review of the benefits of whole body exercise during and after treatment for breast cancer. J Clin Nurs. 2007;6(1):104–21.

Kirshbaum M. Cancer-related fatigue: a review of nursing interventions. Br J Community Nurs. 2010;15(5):214–9.

Kirshbaum M. Pharmacological treatments for fatigue associated with palliative care. Clin J Oncol Nurs. 2011;15(4):438–9.

Kirshbaum M. The benefits of physical exercise for breast cancer patients: a critical review (extended abstract) RCN international nursing research conference, University of Cambridge, Cambridge, U.K. In: 21–24th March; 2004a.

Kirshbaum M. The case for promoting physical exercise in breast cancer care. Nurs Standard (Arts Science). 2005b;19(41):41–8.

Kirshbaum M. Translation to practice: a RCT of an evidenced based booklet targeted at breast care nurses in Britain. Worldviews Evid-Based Nurs. 2008;5(2):60–74. https://doi.org/10.1111/j.1741-6787.2008.00113.x.

Kirshbaum MNY. Disseminating research evidence to breast care nurses: the case of exercise for breast cancer patients. Unpublished PhD thesis. In: University of Manchester; 2004b.

Lanctôt D, Dupuis G, Marcaurell R, Anestin AS, Bali M. The effects of the Bali yoga program (BYP-BC) on reducing psychological symptoms in breast cancer patients receiving chemotherapy: results of a randomized, partially blinded, controlled trial. J Complement Integr Med. 2016;13(4):405–12. https://doi.org/10.1515/jcim-2015-0089.

Leach HJ, Covington KR, Voss C, LeBreton KA, Harden SM, Schuster SR. Effect of group dynamics-based exercise versus personal training in breast cancer survivors. Oncol Nurs Forum. 2019;46(2):185+. https://link.gale.com/apps/doc/A588991408/HRCA?u=ntu&sid=HRCA&xid=b020396e

Lipton BH. The biology of belief: unleashing the power of consciousness, matter and miracles. California: Hay House; 2015.

Lipton BH, Bhaerman S. Spontaneous evolution: our positive future, how to get there from here. California: Hay House; 2009.

Lukas R, Florian S, Frank E, et al. The Research Steering Committee of the European Association for Palliative Care (EAPC) Fatigue in palliative care patients: an EAPC approach. Palliative Medicine. 2008;22:13–32. https://doi.org/10.1177/0269216307085183.

Mao JJ, Styles T, Cheville A, Wolf J, Fernandes S, Farrar JT. Acupuncture for nonpalliative radiation therapy-related fatigue: feasibility study. J Soc Integr Oncol. 2009;7(2):52–8.

Mao H, Mao JJ, Guo M, Cheng K, Wei J, Shen X, Shen X. Effects of infrared laser moxibustion on cancer-related fatigue: a randomized, double-blind, placebo-controlled trial. Cancer. 2016;122(23):3667–72. https://doi.org/10.1002/cncr.30189.

Minton O, Richardson A, Sharpe M, Hotopf M, Stone P. Drug therapy for the management of cancer-related fatigue. Cochrane Database Syst Rev. 2010:CD006704.

Mitchell SA, Beck SL, Hood LE, Moore K, Tanner ER. Putting Evidence Into Practice: Evidence-Based Interventions for Fatigue During and Following Cancer and Its Treatment. Clinical Journal of Oncology Nursing. 2007;11(1):99–113.

Mock V, Burke MB, Sheehan PK, Creaton E, Watson PG, Winningham M, McKinney-Tedder S, Powel L, Liebman M. A nursing rehabilitation program for women with breast cancer receiving adjuvant chemotherapy. Oncol Nurs Forum. 1994;21(5):899–907.

Molassiotis A, Sylt P, Diggins H. The management of cancer-related fatigue after chemotherapy with acupuncture and acupressure: a randomised controlled trial. Complement Ther Med. 2007;15(4):228–37. https://doi.org/10.1016/j.ctim.2006.09.009.

Montgomery GH, Kangas M, David D, Hallquist MN, Green S, Bovbjerg DH, Schnur JB. Fatigue during breast cancer radiotherapy: an initial randomized study of cognitive-behavioral therapy plus hypnosis. Health Psychol. 2009;28(3):317–22. https://doi.org/10.1037/a0013582.

Mücke M, Mochamat M, Cuhls H, Peuckmann-Post V, Minton O, Stone P and Radbrush L. Pharmacological treatments for fatigue associated with palliative care. Cochrane Database Syst Rev 2015: CD006788.

National Comprehensive Cancer Network (NCCN). NCCN guidelines version 2019: cancer-related fatigue; 2019.

National Comprehensive Cancer Network (NCCN). Cancer-related fatigue: NCCN clinical practice guidelines in oncology; 2020. https://www.nccn.org/professionals/physician_gls/pdf/fatigue.pdf

Page BR, Shaw EG, Lu L, et al. Phase ll double blind placebo-controlled randomized study of armodafinil for brain radiation-induced fatigue. Neuro Oncol. 2015;17:1393–401. https://www.ncbi.nlm.nih.gov/pubmed/25972454.

Radbrusch L, Strasser F, Elsner F, et al. Fatigue in palliative care patients: an EAPC approach. Palliative Medicine. 2008;22:13–32.

Rizzo JD, Brouwers M, Hurley P, et al. American Society of Clinical Oncology/American Society of Hematology clinical practice guideline update on the use of epoetin and darbepoetin in adult patients with cancer. J Clin Oncol. 2010;28:4996–5010.

Spathis A, Fife K, Blackhall F, et al. Modafinil for the treatment of fatigue in lung cancer: results of a placebo-controlled, double-blind, randomized trial. J Clin Oncol. 2014;32:1882–8.

Stone P. The measurement, causes and effective management of cancer-related fatigue. Int J Palliat Nurs. 2002;8(3):120–8. https://doi.org/10.12968/ijpn.2002.8.3.10248.

Stricker CT, Drake D, Hoyer KA, Mock V. Evidence-based practice for fatigue management in adults with cancer: exercise as an intervention. Oncol Nurs Forum. 2004;31(5):963–76. https://doi.org/10.1188/04.ONF.963-976.

Tan J, Kirshbaum M, Molasiotis A, Turner C, Moss S, Duddle M, Cheng, HL, Wang CC, Liu X, Zheng S, Waheed. Development and preliminary evaluation of an evidence-based somatic acupressure protocol for the self-management of symptom cluster fatigue, insomnia and depression in breast cancer patients. Charles Darwin University, IAS Rainmaker Grant (unpublished); 2018.

Taso CJ, Lin HS, Lin WL, Chen SM, Huang WT, Chen SW. The effect of yoga exercise on improving depression, anxiety, and fatigue in women with breast cancer: a randomized controlled trial. J Nurs Res. 2014;22(3):155–64. https://doi.org/10.1097/jnr.0000000000000044.

Westbrook D, Kennerley H, Kirk J. An introduction to cognitive behaviour therapy: skills and applications. 2nd ed. London: Sage; 2011.

Winningham ML. Effects of a bicycle ergometry program on functional capacity and feelings of control in women with breast cancer (dissertation abstract). Columbus, OH: Ohio State University; 1983.

Winningham ML, MacVicar MG. The effect of aerobic exercise on patient reports of nausea. Oncol Nurs Forum. 1988;15:447–50.

Yellens SB, Cella DF, Webster K, et al. Measuring fatigue and other anemia-related symptoms with the Functional Assessment of Cancer Therapy (FACT) measurement system. J Pain Symptom Manage. 1997;13:63–74. http://www.ncbi.nlm.nih.gov/pubmed/9095563.

Yennurajalingam S, Frisbee-Hume S, Palmer JL, et al. Reduction of cancer-related fatigue with dexamethasone: a double-blind, randomized, placebo-controlled trial in patients with advanced cancer. J Clin Oncol. 2013;31:3076–82.

Yennurajalingam S, Bruera E. Role of corticosteroids for fatigue in advanced incurable cancer: is it a 'wonder drug' or 'deal with the devil'. Current Opinion in Supportive and Palliative Care 2014;8(4):346–51.

Part II

Philosophy, Evidence, Research and Theoretical Foundations

Philosophy and Theory

5.1 Introduction

We, as *Homo sapiens* who have been living on this awesome planet for over 60,000, are a curious mob. We have striven to gather vital information about our surroundings through observation and experience. This has been the key to our continued survival; one that we should be mindful of as we navigate through what seems to be increasingly difficult times. Through our senses, our large brains and open, loving hearts, we have evolved to decipher and interpret the infinite clues that permeate through our awareness. However, we only process a minuscule part of what is right in front of us. And why is that? you may ask. Well ... there is just too much out there and available to us (Fig. 5.1).

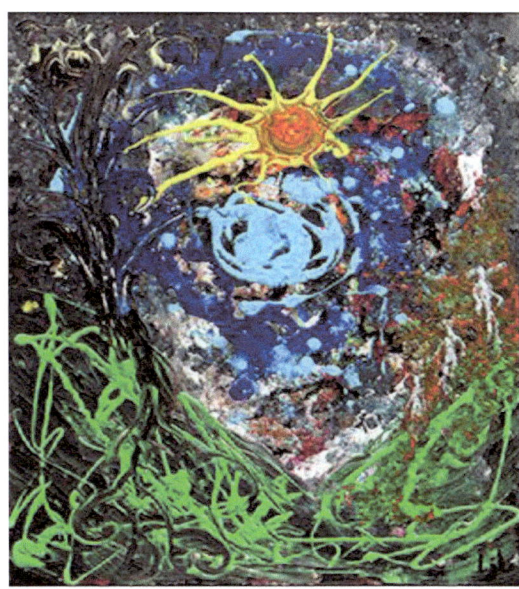

Fig. 5.1 Ayahuasca Night by Laurence James Lucas

M. N. Kirshbaum, *The Joyful Freedom Approach to Cancer-Related Fatigue*,
https://doi.org/10.1007/978-3-030-76932-1_5

Beginning in prehistoric times, we needed to focus on our priorities and develop skills for survival, which we have done. Indigenous people throughout the globe have passed on and retained some of their ancient knowledge, practises and rituals that have enabled humankind to adapt to and survive challenging climatic events, environments and forces of nature throughout history. This is mindboggling to conceptualise. Now that I am living in Australia, I have been trying to grasp the connection that the Indigenous First Nation Australians have with their ancient past, and the time frame of existence for humanity's oldest people and culture. It is very hard to comprehend. From personal experience, I have an inkling of what 60 years on this planet feels like, but 60,000? No way. Time is an abstraction, yet abstraction is timeless.

I can try to understand and begin to have some appreciation of history if I can read and see the path of humanity displayed in a book or museum display, along with milestones of development and achievements. In this way, large amounts of information can be presented in some sort of logical, linear format, and from there I can begin to assemble parts of the puzzle because of the connections that are made between environmental events, emergent advances and displays of artefacts. The lens of the museum display serves to organise and anchor information in one way. Traditional dance and song can be viewed as another lens or artform through which knowledge, stories and sacred wisdoms are interwoven and passed on throughout the ages of the past, present and future.

This chapter will begin with one of the lenses, the philosophy of science, through which various individual and collective perspectives can be used to open up and expand our minds to the wondrous world of knowledge acquisition. You will see that there are many different philosophies, and all represent slightly altered perceptions and versions of *truth*. How can that be? Different truths? Well, yes—that is my view. There can be many truths. I see *truth* as a conclusion that is personal and temporal, whereas *fact*, for me, is a result of objective and empirical processes. I hope you will ponder this a bit … and then proceed with intrigue as we are coming up to a few sections that require some thought about the meaning of *truth* for you and then how best to seek it out through your critical reading of research and perhaps creatively infiltrating the design of your own research study. In all research through discovery within your *truth,* your worldview, should inevitably be aligned with the underlying objectives of your research endeavours, whatever they might be. There will be much more on this later.

In the meantime, I will do my best to introduce many of the confusing and conflicting terms that are used in research methodology books and attempt to provide a clear path through the hazy quagmire of research theory development that is intended to illuminate students, healthcare professionals and interested lay readers. This bridging section is intended to be a foundation to theory appreciation and utilisation within a practice-based healthcare profession such as nursing or social work before introducing and presenting the first version of the energy-creating framework that I have developed initially to help people who suffer from cancer-related fatigue. I will attempt to demystify the theory and language inherent in its purpose, development, critique and utilisation. In this chapter, you will note the deliberate integration of the contributions of philosophy and theory as essential parts of the process to develop a theory based on authentic, humanistic, conscious, systems-based and energy field awareness. Then, in upcoming chapters I will present a selection of relevant and influential theories, models and research that will help situate the framework into its intended philosophical, theoretical and practical context.

5.2   Nursing as a Humanistic 'Modern' Science

The noble profession of Nursing has defined my existence for many, many years. The fundamental caring nature, conceptualised as being both an art and a science, encompassing theory and practice, has remained so central to the way I feel, understand and live my life. The deeper essence of nursing has found its way into my own identity and has been integrated into my teaching and research. However, when I open myself up to the real world of nursing education and practice, the profession of nursing appears to have lost its way over the years. The current state of health care and service user (patient, client and resident) treatment experience is disturbing to me on many levels.

From my professional work and encounters with health care across three continents, more frequently than not, the actions of nurses appear to be subservient to our medical colleagues, who remain the clinical rulers of acute care facilities and governing health authorities. Executive managers are the actual chiefs of most healthcare bodies. This approach does not always serve public needs in an optimum way. Medically trained doctors, surgeons, pathologists, and radiologists are brilliant and literally save lives. I am personally very grateful for having received a couple of life-saving interventions from highly skilled and specialist surgeons in my lifetime so far; I underwent a nephrectomy for suspected cancer when I was 40 years old and then 18 years later, open-heart surgery for an aortic valve replacement. Indeed, truly grateful to be alive and to have the opportunity to write this book for you.

When I try to be objective about the nursing care I have received, well … overall, it could have been better. My impression and therefore, the subjective, non-scientifically measured evidence that was gathered solely through observations of and conservations with nurses as a patient was that nurses did not have an understanding of theory or nursing models. Despite their varied individual personality characteristics, which as a keen observer of humanity kept me a bit entertained, the nurses carried out their routine patient care tasks in a robotic way according to protocols dominated by numerous forms. It seemed that their main reason to interact with me was to complete the necessary and repetitive procedures required to be manually or electronically recorded and 'ticked' as completed. I am not degrading the importance of recording vital signs or fluid balance charts; it was just that I felt that my holistic state of health and wellbeing was not being considered. Where was the human caring element of nursing? From an objective perspective, the psychosocial–spiritual assessments were being overlooked. Despite being a relatively straightforward case, with hardly any complications, I felt sad, lonely, frightened and overwhelmed by the graveness of the surgeries—both times.

It will be fair to say that I would have been oblivious to most of what was going around me due to the pharmaceutically induced dopiness and generalised doziness accompanied with laying in a hospital bed, recovering from major surgery, but I know what I experienced and how I felt. I was aware enough to realise that an important part of nursing care, or rather my view of nursing care, was missing. So, I return to and bring in the inspiring words of Martha E. Rogers:

> *Nursing is a humanistic science dedicated to compassionate concern for maintaining and promoting health, preventing illness and caring for rehabilitating the sick and disabled. Man [Humanity], whom nursing strives to serve, is a unified whole, a synergistic system, who cannot be explained by knowledge of his [their] parts. Sweeping changes taking place throughout the world emphasise life's creativity and challenge the most visionary to foretell the days ahead. The goals of achieving human health and welfare have taken on undreamed-of dimensions as man's [humanity's] earth-bound past merges with his [their] space-directed future.* (Rogers 1970, vii)

These words from the Foreword to Martha E. Rogers' *An Introduction to the Theoretical Basis of Nursing* (Rogers 1970), merged the altruistic, service aspects of nursing with the cosmic, multidimensional and intergalactic perspective that inspired forward-thinking nurses from a long-forgotten era. As a patient and a senior nursing academic, I had hoped that nursing care on medical-surgical units would by now have progressed beyond the mechanistic paradigms of the early twentieth century.

What do I mean by mechanistic? What is a paradigm? What have these nurses done that was so wrong to warrant a mini-rant? Hopefully, by the end of this chapter, you will be a bit wiser and be able to answer these questions in addition to: What is the purpose of a theory? What is a conceptual framework? How does a theoretical model differ from a conceptual one? You are invited to read on.

5.3 Philosophy

If I asked you about your philosophy of life, how would you respond? You might ask a follow-up question such as 'What do you mean'? Who do I follow? I haven't studied philosophy, I don't know about the classical philosophers, I just get on with life'. But I would be interested in hearing about what determines the way you think and act each and every day. I expect it will be different from others whom you meet and even vary between best friends and partners. You might share similar values and assumptions with your family, friends and work colleagues, but your philosophy would be unique, formed by your experiences and genetics (Lipton 2015). I would be asking with an honest intention to get you thinking a bit and certainly not to cause you any discomfort or facial distortions or contortions. We all have a personal philosophy—probably several. Philosophy is all about guiding principles, specifically the principles that frame the way we go about our daily activities and make monumental life-changing decisions.

For the scientist, philosophy relates to the truths underlying scientific knowledge—sometimes this will go beyond the physical and natural world and transcend into the moral or metaphysical realms. What do you think guides the way you approach your life, homelife or work? It is possible you have not taken enough time to ponder this. Once you do, I expect you might find a few discrepancies between what you think might be true, correct and important to you, and what you see being practiced or imposed. Exactly. This can be quite a muddle and be uncomfortably unsettling or lead to acknowledging the discrepancy and go on to full blown disagreement, rebellion or revolution.

But let us not stray too far. I am bringing up philosophy here because I believe it is central to theory development, research and the application of knowledge to practice. In later chapters, I will be presenting an integrated framework that is located in a specific paradigm, incorporates a specific worldview and is based upon a specific epistemology with delineated assumptions. I would like you to appreciate the full scope of my vision so that you can go beyond understanding and utilisation but also take up the invitation to advance this framework towards its full potential towards theory, hopefully, someday.

So, what is philosophy? Philosophy is the study of the nature of knowledge and the reality of its existence. It is 'a study of problems which are ultimate, abstract and general. These problems are concerned with the nature of existence, knowledge, morality, reason and human purpose' (Teichman and Evans 1999). Philosophy can also signify a set of theories of a particular philosopher, a study of the theoretical basis of a branch of knowledge or experience or a theory or attitude that guides one's behaviour (Oxford Concise Dictionary). Philosophers might spend their careers discussing the existential meaning of life analogous to navel-gazing, for example, How did we get here [on Earth]? Was it the work of God, a chance occurrence or something to do with natural selection? What should we do? How do we know what to do? What is there to know?

These questions are very much a part of human existence. And so, demonstrating their very nature, humankind, in the form of self-proclaimed philosophers, has pursued different paths and perspectives that can be organised into different branches of philosophy (see Table 5.1).

It is worth spending some time on this table to appreciate the diversity of philosophy as an academic discipline, one that encompasses an intriguing vastness and expanse of what the human mind may wonder about. Feel free to take some time to contemplate at leisure (Fig. 5.2).

Table 5.1 Branches of philosophy

Metaphysics	Study of the fundamental nature of reality and existence—general theory of reality
Ontology	Study of the theory of being (what is or what exists)
Cosmology	Study of the physical universe
Epistemology	Study of knowledge (ways of knowing, nature of truth and relationship between knowledge and belief)
Logic	Study of principles and methods of reasoning (inference and argument)
Ethics (axiology)	Study of nature values; right and wrong (moral philosophy)
Aesthetics	Study of appreciation of the arts or things beautiful
Philosophy of science	Study of science and scientific practice
Political philosophy	Study of citizen and state

Blackburn (2005) and Teichman and Evan (1999) as cited by McEwen and Willis (2011), p. 6

Fig. 5.2 The Shapeshifters by Laurence James Lucas

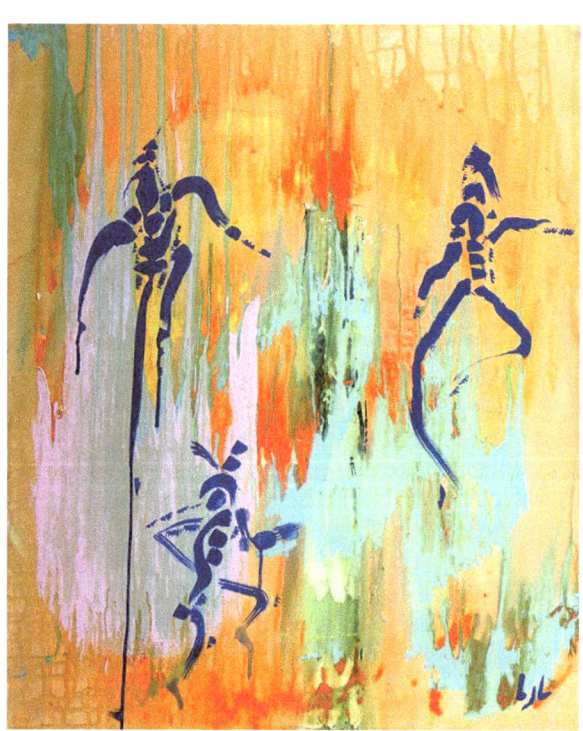

5.4   Scientific Knowledge

The philosophy of science, identified earlier as the study of science and scientific practice, poses questions that attempt to determine *What is scientific knowledge?* and then asks *How do we acquire it?* The research of healthcare professionals mostly falls within this branch although that does not exclude thinking about or integrating perspectives from the other branches. As holistic professionals, we are master integrators of all types of knowledge, experience and skill sets. When we provide direct care or do research that helps our professional colleagues to be more informed about what they do, we draw on biological, chemical, physiological, psychological, sociological and anthropological sources of knowledge.

We are now quite used to the term *evidence-based practice* (see Chap. 6). Most of us in the health field will be aware that *evidence* includes subjective patient and professional perspectives and not necessarily objective, measurable statistically analysed data that are associated with empirical research. As a nurse researcher whose focus is on improving the well-being of people, I value both types of knowledge and strive to integrate multiple perspectives into my work. However, purist philosophers and researchers are likely to align themselves with one of the three main philosophical schools of thought: Rationalism [Rene Descartes 1596–1650 and Baruch Spinoza 1632–1677], Empiricism [Immanuel Kant 1724–1804] and Phenomenology [Edmund Husserl 1859–1938]. This is classic philosophy, worthy of acknowledgement and further reading (Box 5.1).

Box 5.1 Three Main Schools of Thought
Rationalism: deductive, based on reason, rigid (no credence given to individual experience use of mathematical formulae to determine a previously unknown query i.e. If this is X then Y is that …
Empiricism: objective, reductive, verification, deductive, hypothesis testing
Humanistic/Phenomenology: interpretive, descriptive, contextual, holistic

---

For our purposes here, I want to emphasise two points. First, that it is well worth exploring the different schools of philosophical thought so that you can locate where your affinity is placed. This will clarify the characteristics of what is important to you, which is critical to just about everything you do in life, including your approach to research, education and practice. Identifying with a philosophical school will help you determine the type of research that aligns with your interests and affinity toward research approaches, for example qualitative and quantitative/naturistic vs positivistic. Second, it might be obvious and so basic, yet worth a relevant reminder here to highlight the fact that all scientific and interpretative approaches begin with observations, usually of the natural world and its phenomena and interactions. This is the very special place that converges the senses with the word-based cognitive processes where research questions emerge. This is about being present in both our bodies and minds and fully aware of what is going on around us along with a large dollop of curiosity and wonderment. Whatever the discipline or area of research, there will be an infinite number of questions spurred by the inquisitive mind that has tried to process an observation. Let us consider the innocence and openness of a child's perspective—try opening your senses to what is right in front of you and consider, without being too sensible, adult, or rigid and ask: Why is it like that? (child touches, pokes and plays with an object, but it does not do what the child expects and asks,) How can I fix it? (child experiments, moving the object around and different positions) Let us try this and see if it works? (Maybe adding another object to see what would happen).

From my early observations of nursing oncology patients in an acute hospital setting, I used to wonder about so much! I often thought about how basic home comforts were affected. I used to imagine myself in one of the narrow, plastic-covered hospital beds in a room shared with other people with a steady stream of nurses, doctors, pharmacists, physios, occupational therapists and patient visitors, all circulating around while I was clothed in a white hospital gown. This was in the days when the hospital provided open-backed nightwear that was suited for the use of metal bedpans. I have not seen one of those bedpans for a long time, but the basic lack of privacy, noise disturbances and the imposition of other people's problems, distressing episodes and visitors remains in my memory. I spent time thinking, 'How does that affect a person's ability to rest and heal? How can they sleep comfortably in a hospital bed when they would very likely be attached to intravenous monitors and/or be post-surgery and have a painful wound that would hamper movements and body position? How could I sleep on my back (being a side sleeper all my life)?'

Even at the early stage of my professional life, I was interested in finding out about how nurses could support a person's vital healing and well-being therapeutically alongside dominant medical and surgical cancer treatments. This remains the sentinel question for me, which has kept me intellectually occupied and focused for so many years throughout a variety of settings, clinical populations and professional roles.

As I went on to become a more experienced oncology nurse, researcher, educator and Professor of Nursing, I learned quite a bit about the established ways of scientific exploration and investigation as a means of contributing to scientific knowledge. Lesson one is acknowledging that, as in life, there are no shortcuts or free lunches. What exists is a host of research terms that need to be understood. I acknowledge through much experience that learning about research can be particularly challenging and immensely frustrating because just about every book on research methods that I have read or consulted offers slightly different definitions and viewpoints. Before I lead the reader into confusion and the abyss, I will proceed steadily to present quite a few important terms and phrases with the intention of building understanding and appreciation for traditional, evidence-generating research processes.

5.5   Epistemology and Ontology

You might have come across the word *epistemology* before. Hint: it was listed on Table 5.1, towards the earlier part of this chapter as the 'study of the theory of knowledge (ways of knowing, nature of truth and relationship between knowledge and belief)'. This is indeed true. However, I am starting with epistemology because I believe strongly that an early beneficial consideration for any researcher in any discipline or area of study is to identify one's own personal epistemology. This could be done almost instantly, without any influential or corrupting jargon, and that is probably the best way, as it is the purest and surest way to align your internal values and individual belief system to your research approach. It is important because as I have seen with so many colleagues and research students (and in life), if your values align with your actions, your objectives will be achieved with relative ease and enjoyment. However, if you are muddled, distracted, and feel pulled in opposite directions and allegiances, you will struggle with accepting and agreeing with foundational assumptions and processes inherent in your chosen methodology. There will be a hardship, perhaps some distress and possible failure—so let's try to avoid that.

Getting back to epistemology, we can ask: How do we determine what we know? This is about the rationale behind the methodology. Do we ask others to describe their perceptions, opinions and experiences and believe them? This will lead us down the route of qualitative and interpretative research approaches. Or do we set up a study and provide an intervention and then only accept an item of knowledge if it is supported by a statistically significate p value? Do we take a purist and definitive research strategy or design, for example grounded theory, phenomenology, randomised controlled trial or perhaps we appreciate that several types of data collection should be used to provide a more extensive, varied and complete data set that gathers information in different ways from different perspectives, that is mixed method?

Similarly, what do we accept as truth? This is the question posed by *ontology*. McEwen defines ontology as being 'concerned with the study of existence and the nature of reality.' (McEwen 2011, p. 26). I prefer to simplify this by using the powerful word of 'truth'. What do we accept as being real in our perceptions? What do we discard as being false, manipulated or incorrect? When we question: Can there be many and even conflicting truths that correspond to differences in personal experience or perspective, we can decide whether to agree or disagree. Are we prepared to take an inclusive, subjective, accepting and less judgmental ontology that aligns with an integrative, holistic philosophical school of thought? Or are we more inclined to accept only objective, positivistic evidence before confirming a 'truth' or even 'fact'?

Once you have thought about that last paragraph, we can go even further and consider the relationship between knowledge and belief? How much of ourselves should we invest in accepting and integrating the rules and parameters of different schools of thought, which is where I was wanting to lead. To start, a shortcut for professionals is often found in the inherent givens associated with the scope of their particular discipline. Nursing, for example recognises multiple ways of knowing. We value what we observe through the physical assessments that we make on a client, for example blood pressure, temperature, the colour, size, smell and of a wound but also will want to consider what the person has to say about how they feel in regard to their clinical circumstances. Moreover, nurses and nursing research also place great importance on the precise way an intervention is provided. For example, we do not just slap on a clean dressing after ripping off the soiled one. Oh no! We prepare first by checking in with the patient about how they are feeling and explaining what we are planning to do and why, perhaps provide some pain medication, wash our hands, gather the equipment (e.g. clean bandages, cleaning solutions, swabs, gauze and gloves), ensure the patient is comfortable, wash our hands again and proceed according to the latest guidelines to promote the best opportunity for the wound to heal, most probably with some conversation that has a diagnostic or therapeutic intention. These practical actions follow a rational, biological perspective surrounding infection control and wound healing. However, it also integrates the psycho-social perspective of being sensitive to how the person feels overall, responding to the physical task of changing a dressing and offers the opportunity to explore and address any worries or concerns the patient might have.

Also, as a keen student of Martha Rogers, I personally would infuse a more abstract and complex perspective by viewing the dressing change through the lens of her conceptual framework; I would be cognisant of the person's alteration in their physical energy field, meaning, their skin and the existing auric, magnetic and dynamic field. For example: if the patient's primary protective physical barrier [skin] was compromised, I would be attending to the alteration by practicing a strict sterile dressing change. Meanwhile, I would also give some thought to how I would address other physical needs, such as pain relief, use of the toilet and positioning for comfort. The person's cognitive and emotional needs would also need to be met sensitively, efficiently and effectively. The superficial task of a dressing change can become quite sublime, as you will know by now, as the essence of nursing as a humanistic science permeates my mind and infiltrates my being.

5.6 Paradigms

Paradigms are overarching worldviews of beliefs. These global perspectives are made up of closely woven patterns that align with epistemology and ontology. Practically, they are systematic beliefs that provide a platform to organise observations using a lens through which researchers look through when they develop research questions, proposed objectives or hypotheses.

A paradigm is an organising framework that contains concepts, theories, assumptions, beliefs, values and principles that form the way a discipline interprets the subject matter with which it is concerned. It describes work to be done and frames an orientation within which the work will be accomplished. A discipline may have a number of paradigms. The term paradigm is associated with Kuhn's 'Structure of Scientific Revolutions (McEwen 2011, p. 26).

A worldview in my mind is very much a paradigm, just expressed a bit differently:

Worldview is the philosophical frame of reference used by a social or cultural group to describe that group's outlook on and beliefs about reality. (McEwen 2011, p. 26)

I have found that one of the ways to encapsulate the notion of paradigm is to accept that it is intricately aligned with one's profession or specialty. A Rogerian nurse's view would look upon the world and its people through a lens that is concerned with promoting health and integrity of the human energy field thereby preventing illness and would include caring for and rehabilitating the sick and disabled. This focus on the human energy field means that nurses as a homogenous group in terms of their focus and priorities will always be on the needs of the person, whatever the setting. Specialist nurses will modify their focus accordingly. For example, if the setting is in the recovery room post-surgery, every nurse will be bringing in and using all of the supporting elements and resources, such as the monitoring equipment, IV fluids, medications and communication with other healthcare professions to respond to the immediate status and condition of their patient. In contrast, the pharmacist, for example or the physiotherapist will also be attentive to the patient's needs, but their central objective with be aligned with their profession. The pharmacist will be checking and ensuring the availability and safe administration of the drugs and the physio will be more concerned with the positioning of the body and lung inflation.

5.7 Theory

Next up is theory—'Oh no! or 'Hmmm, I'm not sure what you mean'. These are common responses that I have observed firsthand with students, colleagues, friends and acquaintances. I often get the feeling that few people are truly interested although I try to be generous and share my enthusiasm. I realise that most nursing students and registered nurses feel more comfortable hearing about and participating in tangible actions based on objective facts and guidelines that can be used directly in practice. I remember enjoying the very physical and practical side of nursing on mainly surgical units, where morning shifts included making beds, tidying up the bedside, helping people with their hygiene needs, assisting them to move out of bed to a chair or take someone for a walk around the ward, emptying urine and bags with other fluids, attending to IV fluids, changing the dressing, suctioning and so on, while doing a good deal of talking and listening. Each of these tasks is directly informed by an infinite number of theories—it is just that we do not need to consider the theoretical side too much to provide sensitive, informed and safe nursing care. Or do we?

There are many, many, many definitions of theory and several examples of different categorisations. Here are a few as presented by McEwen and Wills (2011):

> … *theory has been described as a systematic explanation of an event in which constructs and concepts are identified and relationships are proposed and predictions made.* (Streubert-Speziale and Carpenter (2006) as cited by McEwen and Wills (2011), p. 22)

> *[Theory is a] creative and rigorous structuring of ideas that project a tentative, purposeful and systematic view of phenomena* (Chinn and Kramer (2008) as cited by McEwen and Will (2011), p. 23)

> *[Theory is] a set of interpretative assumptions, principles or propositions that help explain or guide action* (Young et al. (2001) as cited by McEwen and Will (2011), p. 23)

And then, pulling it all together:

> *Theory refers to a set of logically interrelated concepts, statements, propositions, and definitions, which have been derived from philosophical beliefs of scientific data and from which questions or hypotheses can be deduced, tested and verified. A theory purports to account for or characterise some phenomenon.* (McEwen and Ellis 2011, p. 26).

Fawcett (1984) cites two definitions in her book on conceptual models, which are closely aligned to theories.

> *A theory is a statement that purports to account for or characterise some phenomenon* (Stevens (1979), p. 1 as cited by Fawcett (1984), p. 17)

> *A theory is a provisional explanatory proposition, or set of propositions, concerning some natural phenomena and consisting of symbolic representations of (1) the observed relationships among [measured]events, (2) the mechanisms or structures presumed to underlie such relationships, or (3) inferred relationships and underlying mechanisms intended to account for observed data in the absence of any direct empirical manifestation of the relationships* (Marx (1976), p. 237 as cited by Fawcett (1984), p. 17)

These definitions provide a vague sense of what a theory might be. But despite the intended diligence and precision used to select the most correct terms to explain an abstraction, the end result may still be ambiguous to those who do not have a strong grounding in research. How can someone understand a definition that uses words that are similarly abstract and unfamiliar? I acknowledge that many of the words used to define theory are not normally found or used outside the research area. There remains some work to be done to better understand and I will get on with that, but first let me just say that for me, the last version although longer, is more detailed and closest to the view that I have held for quite a few years. The keywords to note are provisional, proposition and relationships. Kindly accept that a theory is not a fact but an attempt to understand an occurrence [a phenomenon]. Theories are recognisable by being presented as statements that propose some type of unique and novel connection between key players, such as a person and their experience with some aspect of the environment [anything outside of their emotional, psychological or physical body]. Usually, the connection is between articulated concepts that appear within some configuration, such as a representative *model* or a *framework* that emphasises a structure.

In a practice profession such as nursing, there are different types and tiers of theory, which are correspondingly used for different purposes, such as description, explanation and prediction (Fawcett 1984). Theories can also be classified according to their scope and level of abstraction. There are meta, grand, middle range, practice, partial, factor-isolating, factor-relating, situation-relating and situation-producing theories (McEwen 2011). However, I believe that for our purposes, it will be sufficient to distinguish between the grand, middle-range and situation-specific before you get too bored or muddled. *Theoretical Nursing, Development and Process* by Ifaf Ibrahim Meleis (2007) is recommended for further explorations.

Grand theories are the most abstract form of systematic constructs that are formulated from observations and empirical research. Grand theories are inspiring and present huge shifts in perspectives such as Charles Darwin's Theory of Evolution or Karl Marx's Theory and Philosophy. They take a broad view of a discipline and try to explain, often with quite complex terms, an area of central importance. However, grand theories are notoriously difficult to test due to their abstract and their grandiose nature. Rogers' Science of Unitary Human Beings (see Chap. 2) comes close to belonging to this group, and some scholars discuss her contribution as a Grand Theory. However, it probably falls a bit short because of the difficulty in finding testable statements—the ideas are so grand! It is therefore more accurately viewed as a conceptual framework, which for some, is the same. From my investigations, there is no clear consensus.

Moving on, middle-range theories are developed to address specific phenomena or concepts and reflect practice (administrative, clinical or teaching). In sociology, Merton broke some ground in revealing 'the gap between the limited hypotheses of empiricist studies and grand abstract theory of the sort produced by Talcott Parsons' (Clark et al. 1990). He describes middle-range theories as 'theories that lie between the minor but necessary working hypotheses that evolve in abundance in day to day research and the all-inclusive systematic efforts to develop unified theory that will explain all the observed uniformities of social behaviour, organization and social change' (Clark et al. 1990). Merton consistently argued for, and demonstrated the necessity of, this sort of work in a long series of convincing sociological essays in areas such as structural-functional theory and the sociologies of science, deviance, organizations and occupations. Many of the concepts developed in these theories have become part of the basic sociological lexicon.

Examples of middle-range theories would be theories about social support, comfort or community empowerment (Meleis 2007). Situation-specific theories are concerned with a particular population, location or grouping. Smith and Lierhr (2018) have compiled an extensive listing of middle-range theories in nursing, which include references to published articles for each theory. See the Appendix in: https://connect.springerpub.com/content/book/978-0-8261-5992-2/back-matter/app1

5.8 Concepts, Models and Frameworks

Up until now, I have avoided using the most important word of them all—the *concept*. The designation of *concept* can be anything that is important enough to warrant discussion or research. It just depends on the purpose and focus at the time. A concept can be almost anything, with the proviso that you are using the item, emotion, behaviour and event within the realm of research and practice. In philosophy, and therefore when using a research methodology called phenomenology, the central *phenomenon* is more likely to be used. In health care, research examples of *concepts* could be pain, hope, fatigue, person-centred care, trauma, abuse, stress and so on. Concepts can be viewed as building blocks of a framework or conceptual model, as atoms (hydrogen and oxygen) are the building blocks of molecules (H_2O

aka water), except that there will be an infinite amount of literature synthesis from different disciplines and discussion to present to you dear reader.

Models are visual depictions of something larger or more functional, like a model railway or representation of the nature of a relationship between parts of a greater whole or phenomenon. I have never realised this before, but as I am writing this, the existence of the Fashion Model or 'model student' came to mind. So, we do really know about this research term, or do we? Models are hugely variable. In the arena of research that guides practice, models can also be viewed as being empirical, theoretical or conceptual.

McEwen (2011) provides a near-perfect explanation of the term:

> *"Models are graphic or symbolic representations of phenomena that objectively present certain perspectives or points of view about nature, function or both. Models may be theoretical (something not directly observable—expressed in language or mathematical symbols) or empirical (replicas of observable reality—model of an eye, for example)"* (McEwen 2011, p. 26).

Fawcett (1984) wrote an entire book on conceptual models, which was quite authoritative in its day, particularly in American and Canadian schools of nursing, which had a phase of designing entire curricula around one particular model, for example New York University inculcated Martha Rogers' conceptual model. Here Fawcett is determined to 'clarify the confusion between conceptual models and theories seen in contemporary nursing' (p. v11) as there is a very fine line indeed. Several conceptual models are presented and all with the intention of guiding nursing practice and education. As far as the distinction between a conceptual model and a theory, well, theories are more specific throughout—in terms of the definitions of concepts, propositions and testable relationships. Both are quite abstract and overlap depending on their function, that is theories inform research; conceptual models to inform practice and education.

Here, I am trying to build up understanding and appreciation for a framework that I will be introducing later in this book. Concepts of *fatigue, purposeful, expansion, nourishment, connection, belonging* and *fascination* feature in the Energy-restoration Framework, a framework intended as a guiding structure to promote *lifelong self-care* and management of debilitating *fatigue*.

A framework is always about structure and support, whether it is physical as in scaffolding on a building or a climbing frame in a children's playground. Within the research context, a framework provides a logical, not necessarily linear, structure for a defined purpose, most often to justify and guide a research study. Crawford (2020) from an education paradigm provides a thorough chapter that illuminates her view of the difference between a theoretical and a conceptual framework. Most of you will be quite familiar with strategic frameworks that are used in most organisations, such as national health services, universities, charities and businesses to set out a plan for the future. Common features would include a mission statement, pillars or key elements and key performance indicators (KPIs) that act as assessment benchmarks.

For our purpose here, I want to draw your attention to frameworks that have a practice-based intention, where complex and multidimensional factors can be synthesised and ordered in some way to primarily inform practitioners. They could also be characterised as being integrative because their scope goes across several disciplines or worldviews. Furthermore, these types of frameworks are ripe for ongoing, developmental and multi-tiered research to test for content validity, conceptual clarity and theoretical rigour within the 'real world' of practice. The PARHIS (Promoting Action on Research Implementation in Health Services) Framework for Guiding the Implementation of Evidence-based Practice (Rycroft-Malone 2004) is an excellent example originating in the United Kingdom that has been well conceived, developed and presented in the literature.

I hope I have presented some clarity and have not confused the reader too much. It is important to be aware of the terminology, but you do not have to provide your definition of a theory right now. We are moving on …

References

Blackburn S. Oxford Dictionary of philosophy. 2nd ed. New York: Oxford University Press; 2005.

Clark J, Modgil C, Modgil S, editors. Consensus and controversy. New York: Falmer Press; 1990.

Chinn PL, Kramer MK. Theory and nursing: Integrated knowledge development. 7th ed. St Louis: Mosby; 2008.

Crawford L. Conceptual and theoretical frameworks in research. In: Sage; 2020. https://us.sagepub.com/sites/default/files/upm-assets/105274_book_item_105274.pdf.

Fawcett J. Analysis and evaluation of conceptual models. Philadelphia: F.A Davis Company; 1984.

Lipton BH. The biology of belief: unleashing the power of consciousness, matter and miracles. Carlsbad, CA: Hay House; 2015.

Marx MH. Formal theory. In: Marx MH, Goodson FE, editors. Theories in contemporary psychology. 2nd ed. New York: Macmillan; 1976.

McEwen M. Chapter 1: philosophy, science and nursing. In: McEwen W, Mills EM, editors. Theoretical basis for nursing. 3rd ed. Philadelphia: Wolters Kluwer Health/Lippincott Williams and Wilkins; 2011.

McEwen M, Wills EW, editors. Theoretical Basis for Nursing. 3rd ed. Philadelphia: Wolters Kluwer Health/Lippincott Williams and Wilkins; 2011.

Meleis AI. Theoretical nursing: development and progress. 4th ed. Philadelphia: Lippincott Williams & Wilkins; 2007.

Rogers ME. An introduction to the theoretical basis of nursing. Philadelphia: F A Davies; 1970

Rycroft-Malone J. The PARIHS framework—a framework for guiding the implementation of evidence-based practice. J Nurs Care Quality. 2004;19(4):297–304.

Smith MJ, Lierhr RP. Midrange theories for nursing. 4th ed. New York: Springer; 2018.

Stevens BJ. Nursing theory: analysis, application, evaluation. Boston: Little, Brown & Co.; 1979.

Streubert-Speziale HJ, Carpenter DR. Qualitative research in nursing: Advancing the humanistic imperitive. 4th ed. Philiadelphia: Lippincott Williams & Wilkins; 2006.

Teichman J, Evans KC. Philosophy, a Beginner's guide. 3rd ed. Cambridge, MA: Blackwell; 1999.

Young A, Taylor SG, Renpenning KM. Connections: Nursing research, theory and practice. St Louis: Mosby; 2001.

6.1   Introduction

For many years, I was consumed with trying to understand why there was always such a large gap between reading about an advance in knowledge in a published article and then seeing the advantageous outcomes of the study applied directly to people. What was the inherent problem or rather problems of bringing potential clinical benefits to the public? I realised, as you will, that this is a huge area that has fuelled many debates surrounding what is the evidence? When is it considered credible? Who decides what should be put into practice? What are the barriers and limitations that need to be addressed?

Beyond the multitude of empirical research that has been appraised critically by highly authoritative international experts and included in clinical guidelines exists a great expanse of additional knowledge (Fig. 6.1). Here, I am referring to the knowledge that has been gained through small-scale studies where new and potentially valuable interventions are piloted and tested for their effectiveness and feasibility, and where individuals are asked about their personal experiences and understanding. This is the seedbed for future innovations and also, what I believe is sometimes even more important: the ways to integrate and apply new treatments or programs into practice.

This chapter will take you through some of the research literature surrounding the big issues inherent in putting research evidence into practice, clinical effectiveness and also how research findings are broadcast to healthcare professionals, where they can begin to be used and provide direct value to targeted populations.

6.2   Evidence into Practice

6.2.1   Clinical Effectiveness

Providers and consumers of health care regularly express frustration and anger over poor quality service provision, inefficiencies, inequalities and

M. N. Kirshbaum, *The Joyful Freedom Approach to Cancer-Related Fatigue*,
https://doi.org/10.1007/978-3-030-76932-1_6

Fig. 6.1 Create a space
for light by Carey Vail

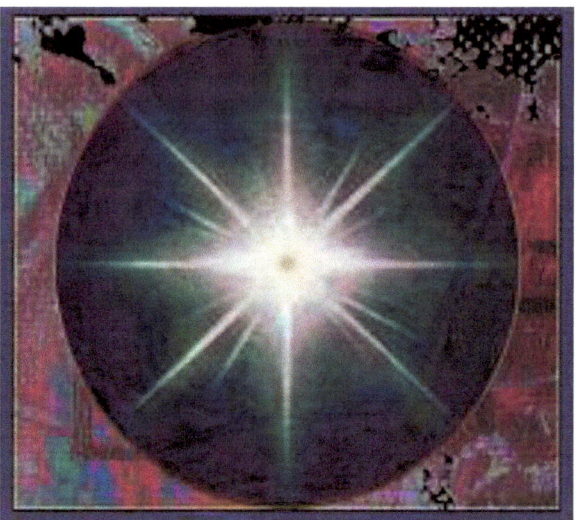

ineffectiveness. The hard reality manifested in such experiences is that the costs of providing even a basic healthcare service are escalating out of control. Privatisation and individual healthcare insurance cannot provide a total solution if we as citizens and healthcare professionals carry out our duty-of-care commitments to improving the health and well-being of all parts of society—to take on our responsibilities with equity and fairness in support of the International Declaration of Human Rights.

This was exacerbated in 2020 when the pandemic of COVID-19 hit most parts of the world. Previously unimaginable actions were taken, as the panic-stricken populations across the planet fought literally for their own survival. Interestingly, we witnessed quite a spectacular irregularity to the usual process of getting clinical research evidence into practice. Vaccines to combat the virus and provide protection for the masses were developed, tested and distributed in record time. Hopefully, by the time this book gets into print, the chaos and extreme loss of life and dignity would have subsided, and we can then begin to integrate what we have just witnessed with the rigours of previous practices, in the interests of ensuring the highest standards of health and well-being possible.

Based on a previous investigation that I conducted, the challenge of dissemination and utilisation of evidence had been well publicised through a series of NHS publications and identified by nurse researchers (NHS Executive 1996a, b, c; NHS Centre for Review and Dissemination 1994; 1999; Cheater and Closs 1997; DiCenso et al. 1998; Titler et al. 1999; Booth et al. 2001; Stevens 2001; Waddell 2002) and they are still very relevant today. *Clinical effectiveness* is a timeless concept that remains at the core of any study or program designed to make a difference to people's health. I have included this section to inform and perhaps remind readers of its importance as a backdrop to presenting the Framework for Energy Restoration. As a framework with such widespread potential, I am determined to do what I can to promote its dissemination and use. Therefore, a brief review of clinical effectiveness and research dissemination methods will follow to bring about my desired outcome of incorporating research evidence into nursing, medical and allied medical practice. To aid understanding of the way in which clinical effectiveness has become a multidisciplinary imperative, some of the terminology used in the literature will be set out briefly into a historical context.

With the publication of a UK government White Paper entitled *A First Class Service: Quality in the NHS* (Department of Health 1998) the imperative directive of 'clinical effectiveness' was declared. The NHS Executive defined clinical effectiveness as:

> *The extent to which specific clinical interventions when deployed in the field for a particular patient or population do what they are intended to do, that is, maintain the health and secure the greatest possible health gain from the available resources* (NHS Executive 1996b, p. 1).

The Royal College of Nursing described clinical effectiveness as:

> *... applying the best knowledge available, derived from research, clinical expertise and patient preferences, to achieve optimum processes and outcomes of care for patients* (RCN 1996).

Both definitions embodied the pervasive drive within the modern NHS at the time to improve the efficiency and quality of healthcare provision; an objective that is relevant to all national healthcare systems the world over. The specific purpose of the *Clinical Effectiveness Initiative* was to provide a national framework that would be used to inform, change and monitor healthcare services within the NHS. All providers of health care, both clinically based professionals and managers, were quick to recognise that there was now added pressure to provide not only an efficient service that made the best use of limited resources but that it was achieved within an evaluative structure centred on the effectiveness of clinical interventions. It was considered imperative to demonstrate that all clinical decisions were based upon the best available evidence from quality research.

The view that a developmental process based on sustained cultural change was underway had been frequently expressed from both nursing (Closs and Cheater 1994; Upton 1999; Kitson 2001) and medical perspectives (Stocking 1992; Oxman et al. 1995; Grol 1997). The NHS Executive was explicit in detailing clinical effectiveness as comprising three distinct steps: (1) obtaining and appraising evidence, (2) implementing the evidence and (3) evaluating the impact of changed practice (NHS Executive 1996b). However, between steps 1 and 2, an implicit stage of crucial instrumental importance in which the evidence obtained is disseminated prior to implementation requires emphasis. Obtaining evidence assumes that two distinct activities, the production and dissemination of research, have been achieved sufficiently. It had been argued that both pursuits inherent in the first component of clinical effectiveness demanded attention from researchers and funding bodies (Newell et al. 1998). It remains to be recognised that dissemination stands in importance alongside the other core components or steps of clinical effectiveness, as it is inextricably linked to knowledge acquisition and the intricacies of behavioural change. Without this recognition, it is unlikely that the complex, multidimensional challenges of achieving clinical effectiveness and integrating beneficial healthcare innovations will ever be met adequately.

6.2.2   Evidence-Based Practice

In the healthcare literature, it is evident that a degree of diversity exists with respect to the definition of evidence. As demonstrated by Le May (1999), a developmental approach to the array of different perspectives can be used to draw out relevant aspects.

The term 'evidence-based medicine' was first defined as 'the conscientious, explicit and judicious use of current best evidence in making decisions about the care of individual patients' (Sackett et al. 1996, p. 71). This definition was succinct and direct. Muir Gray (1997) developed Sackett's definition and included the views of the patient as part of the decision-making process. The concept of 'evidence-based clinical practice' thus emerged as 'an approach to decision-making in which the clinician uses the best evidence available, in consultation with the patient, to decide upon the option which suits the patient best' (Muir Gray 2001, p. 17).

In contributing a health informatics perspective, Booth (1997) extends the definition and writes that:

> *Evidence-based practice is the systematic application of rigorous scientific methods to the evaluation of effectiveness of health care interventions and can be broadened to include such considerations as appropriateness, clinical decision making, economic evaluation, health technology assessment, outcome measurement and risk management.* (Booth 1997, p. 1)

The nursing literature, in an attempt to retain a patient-centred, clinically focused perspective, uses the phrases 'evidence-based practice' and 'evidence-based health care' to refer to all activities informed by research in a way that corresponds loosely to medically focused perspectives such as those mentioned earlier. However, when 'evidence-based nursing' is at issue, the perspective appears to widen further as is demonstrated subsequently.

> *In evidence-based nursing, a nurse has to decide whether evidence is relevant for the particular patient. The incorporation of clinical expertise should be balanced with the risks and benefits of alternative treatments for each patient and should take into account the patient's unique clinical circumstances, including co-morbid conditions and preferences* (DiCenso et al. 1998, p. 38).

Thus, the responsibility of providing patients with clinically effective treatments or interventions is multidimensional. The multidisciplinary variations also serve to indicate that different healthcare professions do not share the same view of the positivist term 'evidence-based care' and might align better with the more inclusive 'research-informed practice' phrase. This is a complicating factor when attempting to define clinical effectiveness in a more generally acceptable way.

6.3   The Problem of Dissemination and Utilisation of Research

In nursing, it follows that the same core components of clinical effectiveness are critically important. A persistent theme in the nursing literature of the past 50 years is the recognition of the difficulty of clinical practitioners to incorporate the findings from empirical research into their practice (Michel and Sneed 1995; Hunt 2001).

Ketefian (1975) is often cited as one of the first nurse investigators to substantiate the observation that, despite the existence of valid and reliable research, most nurses in clinical practice were either unaware of or failed to make use of nursing research findings. In this pioneering study, 87 nurses were surveyed to determine their knowledge and use of research literature surrounding the modes and procedures for taking a patient's temperature. Differences between 'professional nurses' (described by Ketefian as nurses with bachelor's degree from a university) and 'technical nurses' (described by Ketefian as nurses with a lower qualification from a hospital school of nursing) were also analysed. The results indicated that only one nurse in the entire sample demonstrated a familiarity with the guidance derived from the most current research findings. In the discussion Ketefian (1975) reflects:

> A clear picture emerged: The practitioner [nurses in practice settings] was totally unaware of the research literature relative to her practice, or, if she was aware of it, was unable to relate to it or utilize it. There was an apparent isolation of research from practice (p. 91).

From the same study by Ketefian, the observation was made that two distinct sub-cultures existed within nursing. In one group, the researchers produced and disseminated findings to each other, and a second group, the practitioners, lacked awareness of research and consequently did not utilise research findings in their practice. Although it was a pilot study with limited generalisability to all nurses in a clinical setting and insufficient details about the assessment tool, Ketefian's work threw up an array of concerns for nursing practice, education, research and management that still have value today, despite being otherwise out of date. Within the context of the current national evidence-based initiative, Ketefian's concluding remarks provide useful insight.

> … other problems have to do with the existence of barriers to change in organisations where health care is administered and/or delivered. If nurses want to utilise nursing research to improve nursing practice, these barriers need to be understood and contended with—whether they are inherent in organisations or individuals (Ketefian 1975, p. 92).

Further studies have been able to confirm the discrepancy between research and practice within different settings using different methodologies (Horsley et al. 1978; Kirchhoff 1982; Brett 1987; Coyle and Sokop 1990; Michel and Sneed 1995). All have come to similar conclusions. Even the more recent studies conducted after the transfer of nurse education from hospital-based schools to nursing departments within universities has resulted in only slight reductions to the theory–practice gap (Camiah 1997; Rodgers 2000a).

In a recent study that initially included the views of 370 nurses, midwives, health visitors and practice nurses in Wales, Upton (1999) investigated the levels of knowledge and attitudes towards evidence-based practice and clinical effectiveness. Findings from a descriptive postal survey and follow-up interviews reported a generally positive attitude towards research. Respondents frequently made use of evidence-based practice components, such as reviewing their own practice, sharing ideas and information with colleagues and applying information to individual cases.

In a series of four studies (Brett 1987; Coyle and Sokop 1990; Michel and Sneed 1995; Rodgers 2000b), research utilisation amongst hospital nurses was measured using an instrument developed by Haller et al. (1979) within the Conduct and Utilisation of Research Project (CURN) (Horsley et al. 1978). Each study used education interventions to disseminate research evidence to participants who were then assessed by the instrument to produce an outcome score. The determination of the score was standardised and enabled comparison to be made between different studies. The results from Brett (1987), Coyle and Sokop (1990), Michel and Sneed (1995) and Rodgers (2000b) indicated that although there was a pattern of slight improvement, the gap between accumulating research evidence and putting it into clinical practice remained disappointing (Hunt 2001).

In an attempt to disassemble the persistent problem systematically, nurse researchers have documented a long list of reasons as to why nurses do not utilise research in clinical practice (Hunt 1981, 1996, 2001; Rodgers 1994; Hicks 1996; Hicks and Hennessy 1997; Le May et al. 1998; Rolfe 1998; O'Neill and Duffy 2000). A brief summary from Hunt encapsulates the main issues put forward by others and remains representative of contemporary nursing opinion and empirical research literature (Box 6.1).

Box 6.1 Reasons Why Nurses Do Not Utilise Research

1. They [research findings] do not address their problems.
2. They [nurses] do not know about them [research findings].
3. They do not understand them.
4. They do not know how to use them.
5. They do not believe them.
6. They are not allowed to use them.
7. Lack of necessary skills to identify and evaluate relevant research findings.
8. Lack of time to undertake this kind of activity.
9. Lack of access to the right resources.
10. Because they are working within a managerial ethos and culture [and] are expected to devise instant answers

From Hunt 2001, p. 80–81
Included with permission from Wolters Kluwer health Inc. Cancer nursing.

The approach used by Hunt highlighted what she believed to be common themes that would need to be addressed within all empirical work. While Hunt maintained that these themes were grounded in evidence, their impact was not measured quantitatively nor compared in different practice settings amongst nurses with varied levels of research awareness, hence inference and external validity are not substantiated. If research utilisation in nursing and other healthcare professions is to advance, a systematic and robust approach to the identification of barriers is clearly required.

This objective was partially achieved by Funk et al. (1991) who developed and validated an instrument to assess nurses' perceptions of barriers to the utilisation of research findings. The measurement tool, The Barriers and Facilitators to Using Research in Practice Scale, consisted of 29 attitude-type statements about a wide range of potential difficulties related to incorporating research findings into clinical practice (Funk et al. 1987). The scale has been used extensively in practice and research settings in the United Kingdom (Walsh 1997; Dunn et al. 1998; Closs et al. 2000; Parahoo 2000; Kirshbaum et al. 2004), the United States (Rutledge et al. 1998), Sweden (Kajermo et al. 1998) and Australia (Retsas and Nolan 1999). The findings from these similar studies highlight subjectively many of the same difficulties associated with the way research are communicated, the skills of the subjects, the research culture of the organisation and the quality of the research itself.

The main barriers to research utilisation that apply in the United Kingdom such as, not understanding research reports, insufficient time to read the research, not having the authority to change practice (Dunn et al. 1998; Closs et al. 2000) and appear to remain consistent, universal and deeply rooted in nursing culture and practice. A repeated conclusion expressed in the literature was that these barriers cannot be addressed easily or sufficiently in the short term. Multiple, systematic and innovative strategies are still required to remove identified barriers and to strengthen facilitating factors.

The call for both a pragmatic and a systematic approach to the promotion of research utilisation has been expressed by many (Closs and Cheater 1994, Luker and Kendrick 1995, Pryjmachuk 1996, Mulhall et al. 1998) and is an objective that requires sustained political and research action. It appears that for an overall strategy to succeed, a balance of attention and resources would be required to address all three requirements of clinical effectiveness: obtaining evidence, implementing evidence and evaluating the impact of the changed practice. In light of what is already known about the obstacles faced by nurses, ways of improving research synthesis, access and understanding through effective dissemination strategies need to be considered further.

6.3.1 Defining Dissemination

Confusion and alternative interpretations of terminology characterise the body of knowledge referred to as 'research dissemination'. 'Diffusion' and 'dissemination' describe distinctive processes associated with communicating information but are sometimes used interchangeably. This inevitably leads to misunderstanding.

Moreover, the words within the phrases 'dissemination and implementation' and 'dissemination and utilisation' are recognised as being so closely linked that they are commonly discussed as a single concept or activity. Before methods used in dissemination can be reviewed further along in this chapter, an attempt will be made to explain the background to the existing ambiguities and to establish some clear distinctions.

At a basic level, the dissemination of research-based evidence in any academic discipline is generally accepted as involving the movement of information from one point to another. This is most commonly achieved by words on pages of a research article being used as a vehicle to transfer an idea to the mind of the reader. French (1999) expresses this unidirectional view.

> *The process of dissemination [is] the transfer of new information from producers to users* (p. 18).

This definition promotes succinctly the notion of movement between an active 'producer' and a passive 'user'. It is in contrast with another perspective that views dissemination as a multidimensional process:

> *Dissemination is the spread of knowledge from its source to health care practitioners. It includes any special efforts to ensure that practitioners acquire a working acquaintance with that knowledge. Successful dissemination therefore requires both accurate communication from the source and accurate understanding by the recipients* (Lomas and Haynes 1987, p. 77).

This is a more complex view, envisaging the role of the recipient of the information as more than a mere passive absorber. As a multidimensional process, successful dissemination is concerned not only with how a message is transmitted but equally with how the message is received. The phrase 'any special efforts' mentioned by Lomas and Haynes (1987) is a particularly open and non-prescriptive way of expressing that there are potentially many vehicles, methods and strategies to be employed. The crucial point is that the needs of the audience should be an important consideration if successful dissemination of research evidence is the defined objective.

Confusion may arise when the closely related concepts of dissemination and diffusion are discussed within associate health-related disciplines. For example, Green and Johnson (1996) expressed the perception of epidemiologists that diffusion is a process that occurs within the behaviour of populations and that dissemination is focused on groups or individuals. In line with this interpretation, the language of health promotion often uses 'diffusion' in the context of diffusion of ideas into the public domain. This mode of information transfer may be planned strategically at the point of the origin (the sender) yet can be a relatively passive and uncontrolled process as the message moves into new and possibly unknown areas (the receivers). In contrast, evidence-based practice is concerned with the more active form of 'dissemination' of research findings to clinically focused practitioners.

6.4   Review of Dissemination Strategies

As part of my PhD (Kirshbaum 2004a, b), I undertook a systematic review guided by procedures set out by the Centre for Reviews and Dissemination (CRD), University of York (2001), to identify, appraise and synthesise existing literature relevant to the central question: What is known about the effectiveness of methods used to disseminate research evidence to breast care nurses? (Box 6.2) The process can be followed for all systematic reviews, which I hope will be useful to others when they make their own inquires.

Box 6.2 Overview of the Review Process

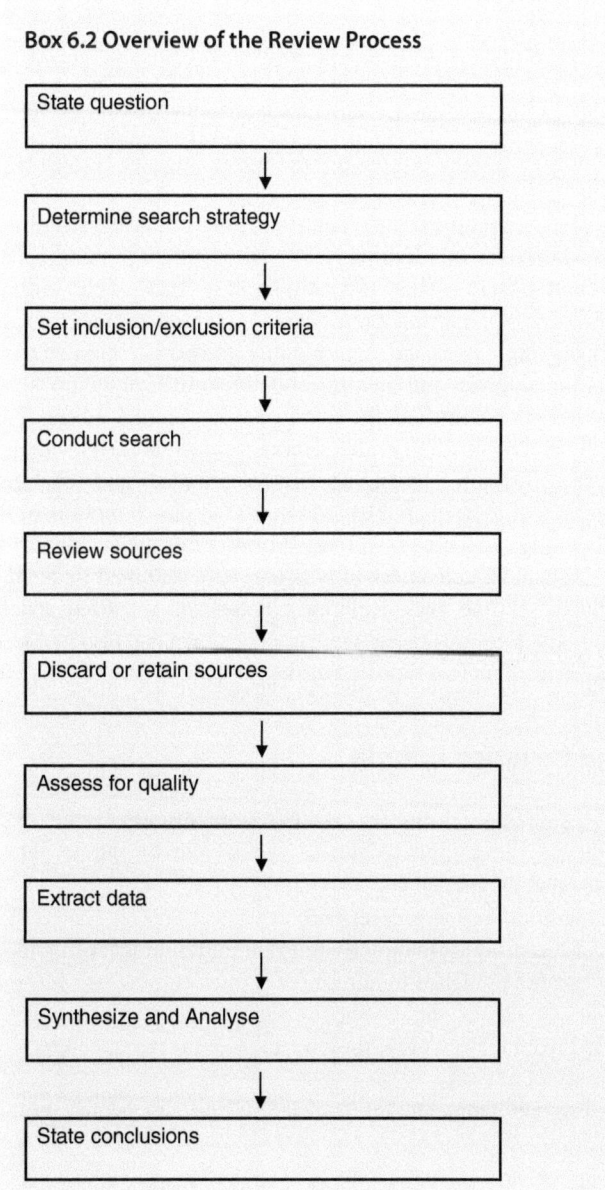

6.4.1   Search Strategy

The PIOC (population, intervention, outcomes and comparison) framework (Richardson et al. 1995) was used to identify core concepts, facets and keywords for searching electronic databases (Box 6.3).

Box 6.3 Components of PIOC framework relevant to the search question

Population	• Breast care nurses, cancer nurses, clinical nurse specialists, nurses.
Intervention	• Research evidence.
Outcomes	• Dissemination methods, evidence-based practice, research utilisation, research evidence, changing clinical practice, changing clinical behaviour.
Comparison	• Not using research evidence.

Multiple search strategies were adopted to identify all the relevant literature in the field. The electronic databases of Medline, CINAHL, British Nursing Index, The Cochrane Library and PsycLit from 1985 to January 2004 were initially accessed for keyword searches of the terms 'breast care nursing/nurses and dissemination methods,' 'cancer nursing/nurses and dissemination methods', 'clinical nurse specialist and dissemination methods' and 'nursing and dissemination methods'. As only three empirical studies were identified, the search was broadened substantially to include the conceptually and contextually related terms: 'information', 'evidence-based practice', 'research utilisation', 'changing clinical practice' and 'changing behaviour'. Individual issues of journals published within the past 6 months of the Journal of Advanced Nursing, Oncology Nursing Forum, European Journal of Oncology Nursing and Clinical Effectiveness in Nursing were searched by hand to allow for publication-database time lags. Reference lists from retrieved articles were reviewed, and potentially relevant studies were tracked down and also included. This produced a snowball effect that was repeated throughout the course of the study.

6.4.2   Inclusion and Exclusion Criteria

Articles were included in the review if they met the following criteria:

• Published in a peer-reviewed journal.
• An explicit research methodology was described.
• Aims and objectives of the study were directly relevant to the subject of methods used to disseminate research evidence to nurses.

Articles were excluded from the review if they were:

• Not written in the English language, as translation services would not be available.

- Methodologically so flawed that findings could not be substantiated (i.e. study design did not address the study's aim).

The decision was also made to not actively seek unpublished 'grey' literature. This was influenced by the comments from experienced researchers who have warned that in circumstances where human and material resources are particularly limited, the time and effort required to locate and review this category of sources would not be warranted (Estabrooks et al. 2003). As the current review was not intended to be a large-scale systematic review or meta-analysis, the advice put forward by Estabrooks et al. was heeded.

6.4.3   Search Results

The search strategy identified a total of 325 titles. Of these, 66 appeared to comply with the inclusion criteria. Full-text articles were then retrieved for a more stringent inspection. Nine studies were retained for the critical review. The majority of papers were excluded because they were not reports of empirical studies nor directly relevant to the focal area of inquiry. Some of these articles expressed interesting insights and applications of theoretical concepts; they were used to inform the researcher of wide-ranging options and possibilities for creative solutions to the research utilisation and evidence-based practice problem. Reports were also excluded due to a lack of sufficient details to determine validity and where the methodological quality was so flawed that conclusions could not be substantiated. One non-English language paper was also excluded.

For more detailed information about the review, please refer to the original dissertation (Kirshbaum 2004a, b). For now, I would just like to mention that three categories of dissemination strategies were investigated for their overall effectiveness to disseminate research evidence to breast care nurses in the United Kingdom: written materials, educational interventions, collaborative and facilitative programs.

The conclusion of the review was that there is universal agreement in both the medical and the nursing literature that providing practitioners with valid, reliable, credible, authoritative, effective and ultimately 'useful' research evidence to inform clinical practice is a highly complex undertaking. There are indeed many varied approaches to communicating clinically relevant information, yet few have been evaluated empirically in nursing populations. Findings from the core studies in the review presented here indicated that:

- Written materials such as information packs and booklets are associated with improvements in specific, topical knowledge and have the potential to have an impact on reported practice.
- Educational methods provided within acute healthcare institutions are varied with some programmes combining several types of educational interventions along with practical applications. However, no generalisations about which programmes are most effective can be made.

- A collaborative and facilitative approach to the dissemination of research evidence may prove to be suitable for nurses, however there are insufficient data about how this is optimally achieved.

References

Booth A. The ScHARR guide to evidence based-practice ScHARR occasional paper no. In: 97/2 University of Sheffield; 1997.

Booth K, Kirshbaum M, Eastwood L, Luker K. Guidance on commissioning cancer services: an investigation of the implications for nursing. Clin Effect Nurs. 2001;5:73–80.

Brett J. Use of nursing practice research findings. Nurs Res. 1987;36(6):344–9.

Camiah S. Utilisation of research in practice and application strategies to raise awareness amongst nurse practitioners: a model for success. J Adv Nurs. 1997;26:1193–202.

Cheater FM, Closs SJ. The effectiveness of methods of dissemination and implementation of clinical guidelines for nursing practice: a selective review. Clin Eff Nurs. 1997;1:4–15.

Closs SJ, Cheater FM. Utilization of nursing research: culture, interest and support. J Adv Nurs. 1994;19:762–73.

Closs SJ, Baum G, Bryar R, Griffiths J, Knight S. Barriers in research implementation in two Yorkshire hospitals. Clin Effect Nurs. 2000;4(1):3–10.

Coyle L, Sokop A. Innovation behaviour among nurses. Nurs Res. 1990;39(3):176–80.

DiCenso A, Cullum N, Ciliska D. Implementing evidence-based nursing: some misconceptions. Evid Based Nurs. 1998;1(2):38–40.

Dunn V, Crichton N, Roe B, Seers K, Williams K. Using research for practice: a U.K. experience of the BARRIERS scale. J Adv Nurs. 1998;26:1203–10.

Estabrooks CA, Floyd JA, Scott-Finlay S, O'Leary KA, Gushta M. Individual determinant of research utilization: a systematic review. J Adv Nurs. 2003;43(5):506–20.

French B. The dissemination of research. In: Mulhall A, Le May A, editors. Nursing research dissemination and implementation. Edinburgh: Churchill Livingston; 1999.

Funk SG, Champagne M, Wiese RA, Tornquist EM. BARRIERS: the barriers to research utilization scale. Appl Nurs Res. 1991;4(1):39–45.

Funk SG, Champagne M, Wiese RA, Tornquist EM. BARRIERS: the barriers to research utilization scale adapted from Crane J, Pelz D and Horsley JA CURN project research utilisation questionnaire Ann Arbor, Michigan;conduct and utilization of research in nursing project, School of Nursing. The University of Michigan; 1987.

Green LW, Johnson J. Dissemination and utilisation of health promotion and disease prevention knowledge: theory, research and experience. Can J Public Health. 1996;87(Suppl 2):S11–S17.

Grol R. Personal paper: beliefs and evidence in changing clinical practice. Br Med J. 1997;315:418–21.

Haller KB, Reynolds MA, Horsley JA. Developing research-based innovation protocols: process, criteria and issues. Res Nurs Health. 1979;2:45–51.

Hicks C. A study of nurses' attitudes towards research: a factor analytic approach. J Adv Nurs. 1996;23:373–9.

Hicks C, Hennessy D. Mixed messages in nursing research: their contribution to the persisting hiatus between evidence and practice. J Adv Nurs. 1997;25(3):595–601.

Horsley JA, Crane J, Bingle JD. Research utilisation as an organisational process. J Nurs Adm. 1978;17:11–8.

Hunt J. Indicators for nursing practice: the use of research findings. J Adv Nurs. 1981;6:189–94.

Hunt J. Barriers to research utilisation. J Adv Nurs. 1996;23:423–5.

Hunt J. Research into practice: the foundation for evidence-based care. Cancer Nurs. 2001;24(2):78–87.

Kajermo KN, Nordstrom G, Krusebrant A, Bjorvell H. Barriers and facilitators of research utiliza-tion as perceived by a group of registered nurses in Sweden. J Adv Nurs. 1998;27:798–807.

Ketefian S. Application of selected nursing research findings into nursing practice. A pilot study. Nurs Res. 1975;24(2):89–92.

Kirchhoff KT. A diffusion survey of coronary precautions. Nurs Res. 1982;31:196–201.

Kirshbaum M. The benefits of physical exercise for breast cancer patients: a critical review (extended abstract) RCN international nursing research conference, University of Cambridge, Cambridge, U.K. In: 21–24th March; 2004a.

Kirshbaum MNY. Disseminating research evidence to breast care nurses: the case of exercise for breast cancer patients. Unpublished PhD thesis. In: University of Manchester; 2004b.

Kirshbaum M, Beaver K, Luker K. Perspectives of breast care nurses on research dissemination and utilisation. Clin Eff Nurs. 2004;8(1):47–58.

Kitson AL. Approaches used to implement research findings into nursing practice. Int J Nurs Pract. 2001;7(6):392–405.

Le May A. Evidence-based practice. London: NT Books, Emap Healthcare; 1999.

Le May A, Mulhall A, Alexander C. Bridging the research-practice gap: exploring the research cultures of practitioners and managers. J Adv Nurs. 1998;28:428–37.

Lomas J, Haynes RB. A taxonomy and critical review of tested strategies for the application of clinical practice recommendations: from 'official' to 'individual' clinical policy. Am J Prev Med. 1987;4:77–94.

Luker KA, Kendrick M. Towards knowledge based practice: an evaluation of a method of dissemi-nation. Int J Nurs Stud. 1995;32(1):59–67.

Michel Y, Sneed NV. Dissemination and use of research findings in nursing practice. J Prof Nurs. 1995;11(5):306–11.

Muir Gray JA. Evidence-based healthcare. Edinburgh: Churchill Livingston; 1997.

Muir Gray JA. Evidence-based healthcare. 2nd ed. Edinburgh: Churchill Livingston; 2001.

Mulhall A, Alexander C, le May A. Appraising the evidence for practice: What do nurses need? Journal of Clinical Effectiveness. 1998;3(2):54–8.

Newell R, Collings L, Forster A, Mackay L. How support teams can develop research activity. Nurs Stand. 1998;12(41):32–3.

NHS Centre for Reviews and Dissemination. Implementing clinical practice guidelines. Effective Health Care Bull. 1994;1(8)

NHS Centre for Reviews and Dissemination. Getting evidence into practice. Effective Health Care Bull. 1999;5(1)

NHS Executive. Guidance for purchasers: improving outcomes in breast cancer. The research evi-dence. London: HMSO; 1996a.

NHS Executive. Promoting clinical effectiveness. A framework for action in and through the NHS. NHSE: Leeds; 1996b.

NHS Executive. Clinical guidelines. Using clinical guidelines to improve patient care within the NHS. NHSE: Leeds; 1996c.

O'Neill AL, Duffy MA. Communicating research and practice knowledge in nursing literature. Nurs Res. 2000;49(4):224–30.

Oxman AD, Thomson MA, Davis DA, Haynes RB. No magic bullets: a systematic review of 102 trials of interventions to improve professional practice. Can Med Assoc J. 1995;153:1423–31.

Parahoo K. Barriers to, and facilitators of research utilisation among nurses in Northern Ireland. J Adv Nurs. 2000;31:89–98.

Pryjmachuk S. Pragmatism and change: some implications for nurses, nurse managers and nurs-ing. J Nurs Manag. 1996;4:201–5.

Retsas A, Nolan M. Barriers to nurses' use of research: an Australian hospital study. Int J Nurs Stud. 1999;36:335–43.

Richardson WS, Wilson MC, Nishikawa J, Hayward RS. The well-built clinical question: a key to evidence-based decisions. ACP J Club. 1995;123:A12–3.

Rodgers S. An exploratory study of research utilisation by nurses in general medical and surgical wards. J Adv Nurs. 1994;20:904–11.

Rodgers SE. A study of the utilisation of research in practice and the influence of education. Nurse Education Today. 2000a;20:279–87.

Rodgers SE. The extent of nursing research utilisation in general medical and surgical wards. J Adv Nurs. 2000b;32(1):182–93.

Rolfe G. The theory practice gap in nursing: From research-based practice to practitioner-based research. J Adv Nurs. 1998;28(3):672–9.

Royal College of Nursing (RCN). Clinical effectiveness: a Royal College of Nursing guide. London: RCN; 1996.

Rutledge DN, Ropka M, Greene PE, Nail L, Mooney KH. Barriers to research utilization for oncology staff nurses and nurse manager/CNS. Oncol Nurs Forum. 1998;25(3):497–506.

Sackett D, Rosenberg W, Haynes RB, Richardson WS. Evidence-based medicine: what it is, what it isn't. Br Med J. 1996;312:71–2.

Stevens KR. The truth. In: the whole truth about EBP and RCTs (editorial) Online Journal of Knowledge Synthesis for Nursing September 20th; 2001. www.stti.iupui.edu/library/ojksn/e_truth_ebp.html.

Stocking B. Promoting change in clinical care. Qual Health Care. 1992;1:56–60.

Titler MG, Mentes JC, Rakel BA, Abbott L, Baumler S. From book to bedside: putting evidence to use in the care of the elderly. J Qual Improv. 1999;25(10):545–56.

Upton D. Attitudes towards, and knowledge of, clinical effectiveness in nurses, midwives, practice nurses and health visitors. J Adv Nurs. 1999;29(4):885–93.

Waddell C. So much research evidence, so little dissemination and uptake: mixing the useful with the pleasing. Evidence Based Nursing. 2002;5:38–40.

Walsh M. How nurses perceive barriers to research implementation. Nurs Stand. 1997;11(29):34–9.

Research in Practice

7

7.1   An Educational Intervention for Physical Exercise in Breast Cancer Care

Based on the conclusions of the review of dissemination methods, a randomised controlled study was devised (Kirshbaum 2008). This followed the publication of the resultant conceptual framework for research dissemination (Kirshbaum 2005a) and an article on promoting physical exercise in breast cancer care (Kirshbaum 2005b). This main randomised study challenged the evidence surrounding the effectiveness of written education materials (Fig. 7.1). The study evaluated the effect of a target booklet, Exercise and Breast Cancer: A Booklet for Breast-Care Nurses, on

Fig. 7.1 Manton Dam, Northern Territory photo by Marilynne N Kirshbaum

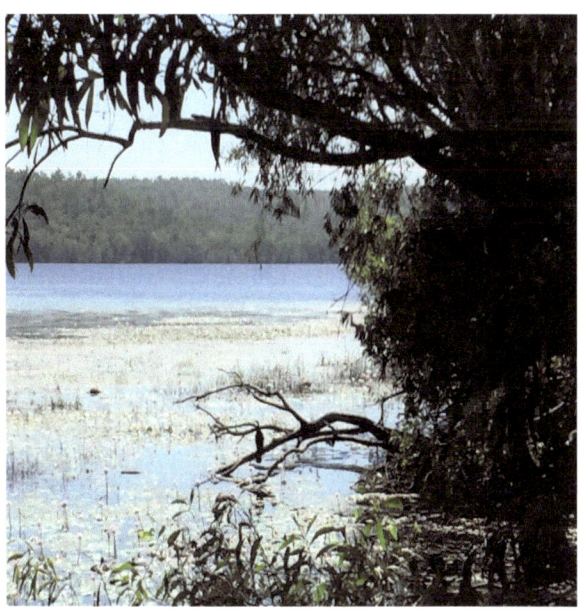

© Springer Nature Switzerland AG 2021
M. N. Kirshbaum, *The Joyful Freedom Approach to Cancer-Related Fatigue*,
https://doi.org/10.1007/978-3-030-76932-1_7

changes in knowledge, reported practice and attitudes of breast care nurses (Kirshbaum 2008). This study of 92 breast care nurses working in 63 hospitals in the United Kingdom (overall response rate of 69%) showed not only a successful choice of format for disseminating knowledge about the benefits of exercise to reducing cancer-related fatigue but also that nurse researchers can be effective change agents in promoting effective, non-medical interventions.

The intervention was an evidence-based booklet, targeted to the audience of specialist breast care nurses. Therefore, professional terminology and the inclusion of the results of a full systematic review of the benefits of exercise for breast cancer patients was integrated along with information about specific psycho-social and physical needs, the barriers and limitations to moderate, physical and aerobic exercise for this client group and recommendations of how to overcome some of the identified barriers and limitations.

The resultant randomised controlled study demonstrated a statistically significant increase in knowledge due to robust variables such as promotion of health, promotion of exercise and understanding how exercise can reduce cancer-related fatigue. The study also showed that an example of an evidence-based printed material, such as an information booklet, can be used as an effective research dissemination method when developed to align with the needs, values and context of a targeted audience.

7.2   Understanding the Meaning of Fatigue at the End of Life: An Ethnoscience Study

7.2.1   Introduction

In the continuing quest to understand the complexity of cancer-related fatigue through empirical research, I joined with researchers from four other countries and used an approach called Ethnoscience, which gave prominence to the words people used to describe their fatigue (Kirshbaum et al. 2010; Kirshbaum et al. 2012; Olson et al. 2015). We went back to a troubling problem historically plaguing researchers working within this area of fatigue management.

[the following excerpts are used with permission from Elsevier and available on Science Direct, originally published in the European Journal of Oncology Nursing]

For example, Bartley and Chute (1947), two of the earliest fatigue researchers, described fatigue as an indicator that the body lacked resources to cope with physical demands placed upon it. Years later, Grandjean (1968) proposed a biofeedback process that linked fatigue, consciousness, perception and thinking. Grandjean's work formed a foundation for the most recent studies of fatigue. Piper used Grandjean's ideas to develop the Integrated Fatigue Model (1987), which is comprised of four fatigue manifestations (perception, physiological, biochemical and behavioural) surrounded by 13 types of 'patterns' that influence the perception of fatigue and its clinical manifestation.

The Psychobiological-Entropy Hypothesis postulated by Winningham emphasized an approach based upon balancing restorative rest with restorative activity

(Nail 1997). Kralik et al. (2005) have described fatigue as a 'multi-dimensional and complex phenomenon that affects physical, cognitive, emotional and social functioning' (p. 378), which concurs with the literature (Piper et al. 1987; Richardson 1995; Krupp and Christodoulou 2001; Ameringer and Smith 2011). A more recent approach to the management of fatigue in cancer care has been to view and attempt to treat multiple symptoms simultaneously as a cluster (Dodd et al. 2001; Barsevick 2007).

This study is built upon different conceptualisations of fatigue based in stress theory (Selye 1950, 1956, 1971; Aistars 1987; Cameron 1997; Glaus 1998). Using this approach, Olson conducted an extensive review of the literature and a series of qualitative studies in populations who experienced fatigue for different reasons and proposed that fatigue was a behavioural marker for the inability to adapt to stressors associated with advanced chronic disease and treatment (Olson 2007; Olson et al. 2007, 2008). These stressors reduced the inability to adapt by causing a decline in cognitive functioning, muscle endurance, sleep quality, social interactions, and an increase in emotional reactivity. Olson distinguished between tiredness, fatigue and exhaustion on the basis of changes in these five areas (Olson 2007). For example, individuals with fatigue reported difficulty concentrating, and individuals with exhaustion reported confusion.

7.2.2   The Study

Our team was comprised of researchers from Canada, Italy, Thailand, England and Sweden. We were interested in the idea that in addition to stressors associated with disease and treatment, the manifestations of fatigue are also influenced by the meanings we attach to fatigue and that these meanings are socially constructed. This idea is supported by the work of Kleinman et al. (2006) who argue that the perceptions associated with illness are influenced by social spheres of life such as gender, family, age, socioeconomic status, geographical location and occupation.

This study replicated the ground-breaking work of Olson et al. (2007) across several countries, which enabled us to dive down into different social sphere in an attempt to: identify the behavioural patterns that distinguish fatigue from tiredness and exhaustion and provide conceptual definition of tiredness, fatigue and exhaustion.

I led the research team in the north of England which took place in an established hospice in the suburbs of a large city. Informants needed to be in the palliative stage of any illness; have self-reported experience of tiredness, fatigue or exhaustion and have enough energy to be interviewed for 45 min at a time.

Nine participants, eight of whom had cancer, were interviewed twice using an ethnoscience design involving a card sort process described by Spradley (1979). Index cards were used to generate keywords and phrases used by participants to recount the meaning and patterns inherent in their fatigue. This formed the basis for our data collection which was analysed by ethnographic content analysis (Altheide 1999; Altheide 2004). A Taxonomy of Fatigue (Table 7.1) was proposed which

Table 7.1 Taxonomy of fatigue: comparing tiredness, fatigue and exhaustion

Segregates	Sub-segregates	Domains		
		Tiredness	Fatigue	Exhaustion
The mental challenge	Emotional effect of decline	Mood is variable, dependent on type and level of activity	Characterized by annoyance, frustration, worry	Sense of giving in (to sleep, to health)
	Cognitive realisation of decline	Attributable to an identifiable cause	Day to day struggle (but still benefitting from palliative treatments and medications)	Noticeable decline
	Mental tenacity	Able to plan and complete activities	Realise that sometimes they cannot push themselves—there is not enough energy to complete task	Little indication of 'pushing self' and wanting to do more
The physical challenge	Limitations in leisure activity	Able to continue activity	Continues activity with imposed limitations energy to complete task 'Can't do what I want to do'	Does not consider doing activity (unless has large amount of support)
	Limitations in functional roles	Able to continue activity	Continues activity with imposed limitations	Does not consider doing activity (unless has large amount of support)
	Re-patterning routines	Able to adjust lifestyle	Plans and re-patterns lifestyle but sometimes gets 'caught out' cannot finish what was planned) Can describe a "pattern of liveliness to exhaustion"	Does not attempt to re-pattern gives in to sleep

Reprinted with permission from Elsevier, Kirshbaum et al. (2012)

compared tiredness, fatigue and exhaustion (domains) according to mental and physical challenges (as segregates) and six divisions (sub-segregates).

I would urge you to access the original article for more details about the research design, analysis and findings of the England study (Kirshbaum et al. 2012) and also the corresponding publications of the cross-cultural, international team to obtain the full impact of this work (Graffigna et al. 2011; Barello et al. 2013; Pongthavornkamol et al. 2012; Kirshbaum et al. 2012; Olson 2007). In the meantime, I can report that the differences between the countries were subtle and supported the proposition that 'meanings attached to symptoms are socially constructed … they raise the important issue of thinking about how the differences in meaning could be built into interventions in ways that are appropriate to one's social context. The participants in this [English] study were proud of their tenacity and the ways in which they were solving their functional challenges. They were distressed by situations in which their abilities were not recognised or accommodated. Participants in this study seemed to want to play an active role in ongoing daily activity and did not perceive any cognitive limitations in doing so.'

References

Aistars J. Fatigue in the cancer patient: a conceptual approach to a clinical problem. Oncol Nurs Forum. 1987;14:25–9.

Altheide DL. Qualitative media analysis. In: Bryman A, Burgess RG, editors. Qualitative Research (volume 2). Thousand Oaks, California: Sage; 1999. p. 235–55.

Altheide DL. Ethnographic content analysis. In: Lewis-Beck MS, Bryman A, Liao TF, editors. The sage encyclopedia of social science research methods. Thousand Oaks, California: Sage; 2004. p. 325–6.

Ameringer S, Smith WR. Emerging biobehavioural factors of fatigue in sickle cell disease. J Nurs Scholarsh. 2011;43:22–9.

Barello S, Lamiani G, Graffigna G, Luciani A, Vegni E, Saita E, Olson K, Bosio C. How patients experience and give meaning to their cancer-related fatigue? A qualitative research in the Italian context. Int J Soc Sci Stud. 2013;1(2) https://doi.org/10.11114/ijsss.v1i1.44.

Barsevick AM. The elusive concept of the symptom cluster. Oncol Nurs Forum. 2007;34:971–80.

Bartley S, Chute E. Fatigue and impairment in man. New York: McGraw Hill; 1947.

Cameron C. A theory of fatigue. Ergonomics. 1997;16:633–48.

Dodd M, Miaskowski C, Paul SM. Symptom clusters and their effect on the functional status of patients with cancer. Oncol Nurs Forum. 2001;28:465–70.

Glaus A. Fatigue in patients with cancer. Berlin: Springer; 1998.

Graffigna G, Vegni E, Barrello S, Olson K, Bosio CA. Studying the social construction of cancer-related fatigue experience: the heuristic value of Ethnoscience. Patient Educ Couns. 2011;82:402–9.

Grandjean E. Fatigue: its physiological and psychological significance. Ergonomics. 1968;11:427–36.

Kirshbaum M. A conceptual framework for targeting research dissemination interventions to meet the needs of breast cancer patients in the United Kingdom. (Published conference abstract). Oncol Nurs Forum. 2005a;32(1):164

Kirshbaum M. The case for promoting physical exercise in breast cancer care. Nurs Standard (Arts Science). 2005b;19(41):41–8.

Kirshbaum M. Translation to practice: a RCT of an evidenced based booklet targeted at breast care nurses in Britain. Worldviews Evid-Based Nurs. 2008;5(2):60–74. https://doi.org/10.1111/j.1741-6787.2008.00113.x.

Kirshbaum M. Cancer related fatigue: a review of nursing interventions. Br J Community Nurs. 2010;5(5):220–4. https://doi.org/10.12968/bjcn.2010.15.5.47945.

Kirshbaum M, Olson K, Pongthavornkamol K, Graffigna. Understanding the meaning of fatigue at the end of life: an ethnoscience study. Eur J Oncol Nurs. 2012;17:146–53. https://doi.org/10.1016/j.ejon.2012.04.007.

Kleinman A, Eisenberg L, Good B. Culture, illness, and care: clinical lessons from anthropologic and cross cultural research. Focus. 2006;4:140–9.

Kralik D, Telford K, Price K, Koch T. Women experiences of fatigue in chronic illness. J Adv Nurs. 2005;52:372–80.

Krupp LB, Christodoulou C. Fatigue in multiple sclerosis. Curr Neurol Neurosci Rep. 2001;1:294–8.

Nail L. Fatigue. In: Groenwald SL, Frogge MH, Goodman M, Yarbro C, editors. Cancer nursing: principles and practices. 4th ed. Boston: Jones and Barlett; 1997. p. 640–54.

Olson K. A new way of thinking about fatigue: a reconceptualization. Oncol Nurs Forum. 2007;34:93–9. https://doi.org/10.1188/07.ONF.93-99.

Olson K, Turner R, Courneya KS, Field C, Man G, Cree M. Possible links between behavioral and physiological indices of tiredness, fatigue and exhaustion in advanced cancer. Support Cancer Care. 2008;16:241–9.

Olson K, Krawchuk A, Quddusi T. Fatigue in individuals with advanced cancer in active treatment and palliative settings. Cancer Nurs. 2015;30:E1–E10.

Piper BF, Lindsey AM, Dodd M. Fatigue mechanisms in cancer patients: developing nursing theory. Oncol Nurs Forum. 1987;14:17–23.

Pongthavornkamol K, Olson K, Soparatanapaisarn N, Chatchaisucha S, Kamkhon A, Potaros, Kirshbaum M, Graffigna G. Comparing the meanings of fatigue in individuals with cancer in Thailand and Canada. Cancer Nurs. 2012;35(5):E1–9. https://doi.org/10.1097/NCC.0b013e3182331a7c.

Richardson A. Fatigue in cancer patients: a review of the literature. Eur J Cancer Care. 1995;4:20–32.

Selye H. Stress and the general adaptation syndrome. Br Med J. 1950;4667:1383–92.

Selye H. The stress of life. New York: McGraw Hill; 1956.

Selye H. Hormones and resistance (volume 1). New York: Springer; 1971.

Spradley JP. The ethnographic interview. New York: Holt, Rinehart & Winston; 1979.

Theoretical Musings: Towards Energy Restoration

8

8.1 Introduction

We can live our lives according to regimented routines, ordered and scheduled to achieve maximum outcomes and achievements and seemingly do just fine for our entire lifespan. Most of us will have our ups and downs and deal with the joys and challenges that fill the years from birth to eventual death. During this time, we get to know ourselves well too. For me, I know that every so often I stumble upon some idea, perspective or person that fills me with immense inspiration (Fig. 8.1). This feeling can be extremely intense and consume much of my inner thoughts and

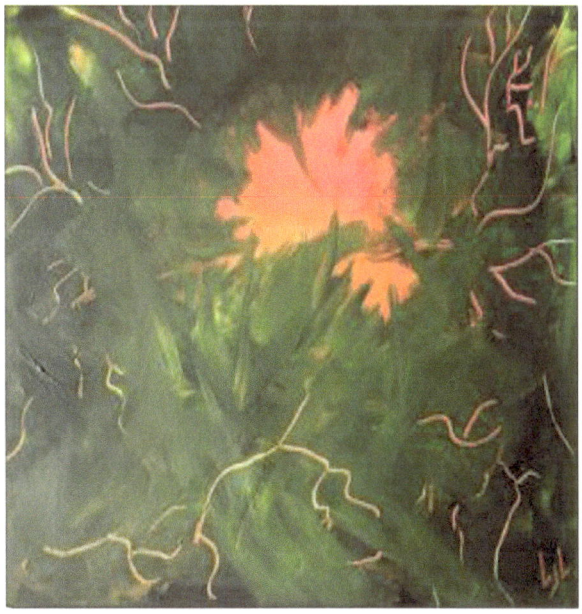

Fig. 8.1 In the Heart of the Forest by Laurence James Lucas

© Springer Nature Switzerland AG 2021
M. N. Kirshbaum, *The Joyful Freedom Approach to Cancer-Related Fatigue*,
https://doi.org/10.1007/978-3-030-76932-1_8

contemplations during wakeful and slumber time hours, not just for a few days but for years!

I was in Yorkshire, England, and I had completed the UK contribution to a multinational ethnoscience study on fatigue (Kirshbaum et al. 2012) at the local hospice there. Concurrently, and for several years during this period, I had the privilege of giving regular talks to women who had breast cancer through the charity Breast Cancer Care. This was mostly around the content of understanding cancer-related fatigue which progressed to practical and evidence-based advice that could help. The most effective, research-based self-care recommendation at that time, and still remains, is regular moderate aerobic exercise. Other advice and helpful recommendations were gathered and shared from clinical guidelines, such as the NCCN (2020), published articles and personal experiences, which included the mention of energy conservation, Tai Chi and Qigong, meditation, sleep management/hygiene, Cognitive Behaviour Therapy (CBT), analysis of negative emotions, communion with nature, a range of holistic complementary therapies and really anything else that the women in the various groups had tried and found helpful and worthy of discussing with others. For these sessions, I remember keeping an open mind about what could be helpful and never disregarded or strongly refuted contributions from participants. Just because there may have been insufficient statistical evidence to support a particular approach or specific activity because the meta-analyses of large-scale Randomised Controlled Trial (RCT) had not made a definitive conclusion, did not necessarily mean that the intervention or approach could not be beneficial. Importantly, it was a clear indication that more research was needed.

Indeed, more research was and is still needed. Aside from regular moderate aerobic exercise and a few articles in support of the structured therapeutic approach provided through CBT, there was not much else that had been substantiated in the research literature, guidelines or systematic reviews. There was still a knowledge gap between what these women were doing and what was evidenced as being effective. I was driven to find a way through to answer a BIG question. However, it was not necessary to do with conducting many studies on each of the proposed (or infinite) interventions or approaches. I wanted to know why some interventions or approaches were so helpful to some women and not others. Practically, it made some sense due to the variations between people. Not all of us are exercise enthusiasts or feel confident or disciplined enough to meditate on their own; we have different perceptions about what constitutes 'soothing' music, and some people really love 'Who done it?' crime mysteries. Where am I going with this? Well, as before, I came across an inspiring article, and again, I was drawn into a different paradigm—an alternative way of approaching cancer-related fatigue.

8.2   Attention Restoration Theory

It occurred to me that I was looking for some kind of practical framework. In other words, I wanted to find some type of structure that could help me understand and ultimately provide a practical guide for people to manage and address their own fatigue, not just for people who have cancer but for everyone who identified with having less than optimal energy levels. Was that unreasonable? Well, I found what I was looking for, but with a few missing parts.

My quest was fulfilled and invigorated through reading *The Restorative Benefits of Nature: Toward an Integrative Framework* (Kaplan 1995). In this article, Kaplan draws on his Attention Restorative Theory (ART), which led me into another inquisitive dimension and yearning to delve in further to find out more. Furthermore, I discovered that a nurse had also come across Kaplan's work too and had started to apply it to people who had cancer (Cimprich 1992, 1993), but that was a very long time ago. I was clearly on to something here.

Professor Stephen Kaplan worked closely with his wife Professor Rachel Kaplan, also an esteemed academic based at the University of Michigan, USA. Together and apart, they contributed a sizeable body of knowledge about mental fatigue that merged environmental perspectives with psychology and social community-based approaches that included three books: *Humanscape: Environments for People* (Kaplan and Kaplan 1978), *Cognition and Environment: Functioning in an Uncertain World* (Kaplan and Kaplan 1982) and *Fostering Reasonableness: Supportive Environments for Bringing Out Our Best* (Kaplan and Basu 2015).

The backdrop to Stephen Kaplan's ART (Kaplan 1995, 2001; Sullivan 2015) considered how we take in information—this was found to have a significant effect on mental fatigue. Kaplan drew upon the work of William James (1892) who first wrote about *voluntary attention*, 'employed when something did not in itself attract attention, but when it was important to attend nonetheless' (Kaplan 1995, p. 169). Kaplan took the concepts of *intention* and *effort,* which are part of the abstract discussion, and began to present the difference between *directed attention* and *involuntary attention.* The theory then goes on to describe the four overarching properties, referred to as *attributes,* as remedies for the fatigue caused by directed attention. I will explain …

Throughout our day, we will often find ourselves doing activities that require effort, concentration and maintaining focus, whether we like it or not. To enable us to focus when our intention is weak or challenged in some way, we will have to ignore peripheral stimuli and thoughts. This characteristic of attention is called *directed attention* and it causes *directed attention fatigue (DAF).* We can all relate to this immediately—this is exactly what we do so much of the time when we are at work: reading and responding to emails, participating in meetings, listening to a lecture or webinar, providing a treatment or therapeutic session, fixing a leak in a water pipe and so on …

DAF pertains to the activities performed in most jobs and the responsibilities and tasks that are required. Our numerous and diverse interpersonal relationships also fall into this grouping. For example, DAF occurs when you are listening carefully to a softly spoken person when there is lots of background noise. It requires effort, even if you are interested in what the other person is saying. After a while, you might not even realise it, but the encounter would have drained you of some energy and caused you to feel fatigued at the end of the day, or when you have stopped pumping adrenaline or caffeine into your system in order to get through. Like stress,

DAF is cumulative; it builds and builds until you can no longer go on—you need to stop and collapse in a heap of frustration, exhaustion or both. Kaplan presents a full discussion of the importance of *directed attention* and the consequences of DAF in terms of ineffectiveness, human error and serious accidents; the theoretical components are further delineated under the headings of inhibition and affect, fragility, perception, thought, action and feeling (Kaplan 1995).

Thankfully, we as human beings have within ourselves, whatever our circumstances, opportunities to participate or take delight in activities that are associated with *involuntary attention*. These activities are characterized by fascination, innate interest, curiosity and exploration—they are effortless and do not result in fatigue; they are *restorative*. Sleep is surely restorative as is a simple change in environment but may not offer enough or the right kind of restorative energy. Furthermore, insomnia can also feature in this space of DAF where there is increased stimulation and preceptory overload.

According to Kaplan, *fascination* is at the core of *involuntary attention*, and is central to the restorative experience, but is limiting for recovering from DAF. So, in addition, three other attributes of the restorative experience are identified: *being away, extent* and *compatibility*.

In respect to the man who is now at rest from a long-standing illness, I present to you Kaplan's description of the four attributes in his own words, rather than risk misinterpretation of his sensitive observation and brilliance.

The Restoration Experience
The restoration of effectiveness is at the mercy of recovery from directed attention fatigue … There are many sources and types of fascination. Some of these derive from process. For instance, otherwise normal individuals have been reported to rouse themselves out of bed at an early hour in hopes of catching a glimpse of a small, feathered animal whose identity is uncertain. Likewise, many are addicted to books in which the identification of the guilty party is difficult but not impossible to predict, and generally is not resolved until the end, even though far more efficient ways to transmit the same information are surely available. Predicting despite uncertainty as practised by gamblers provides another example of process fascination.

Fascination can also come from content. As previously noted, wild animals and caves are among the many contents that do not require directed attention. In some cases extremes of size lend to the fascination of objects or settings. Fascination can also derive from extremes along a 'soft-hard' dimension. Thus, there is the 'hard' fascination of watching auto racing and 'soft' fascination of walking in a natural setting. Soft fascination-characteristic of certain natural settings-has a special advantage in terms of providing an opportunity for reflection, which can further enhance the benefits of recovering from directed fatigue (Kaplan 1995, p. 172)

Being away, at least in principle, frees one from mental activity that requires directed attention support to keep going. In fact, people often use 'getting away' as a shorthand for going to a restorative place. But continuing to struggle with the old thoughts in a new setting is unlikely to be restorative. Clearly being away involves a conceptual rather than physical transformation. A new or different environment, while potentially helpful, is not essential. A change in the direction of one's gaze, or even an old environment viewed in a new way can provide the necessary conceptual shift.

*   The environment must have extent. It must, in other words, be rich enough and coherent enough so that it constitutes a whole other world. An endless stream of stimuli both fascinating and different from the usual would not qualify as a restorative environment for two reasons. First, lacking extent, it does not qualify as an environment, but merely an unrelated collection of impressions. And second, a restorative environment must be of sufficient scope to engage the mind. It must provide enough to see, experience and think about so that it takes up a substantial portion of the available room in own's head.*

*   There should be compatibility between the environment and one's purposes and inclinations. In other words, the setting must fit what one is trying to do and what one would like to do ... in a compatible environment one carries out one's activities smoothly and without struggle. There is no need to second guess or to keep a close eye on one's own behaviour.* (Kaplan 1995, p. 173)

Reprinted from The Restorative Benefits of Nature: Toward an Integrative Framework, Stephen Kaplan Journal of Environmental Psychology 15:172,173. 1995 with permission from Elsevier.

When I first read about Kaplan's description of *directed* and *involuntary attention* (Kaplan 1995), I was captivated. The notion of DAF and the attributes of attention restorative activities made complete sense to me in relation to my own fluctuating energy levels. I started to experiment on myself and log my daily activities, energy levels (on a scale of 1–5) and any direct action that I took to enliven and restore myself to a preferable higher energy state once I noticed I was feeling depleted.

The objective of my personal experiential approach was to internalise the attributes presented by Kaplan and try to deepen and broaden my understanding of them, including the lateral nuances and associations. For example, what did Kaplan mean by 'extent'? He wrote about the notion of coherence and alignment. I was assuming that this attribute had something to do with values and internalised behaviour. So, if an activity conforms to how one usually thinks, behaves and acts, without a huge learning curve or requirement to plod on outside of one's comfort zone, then energy would surely be conserved. On a slightly deeper level, I am also including the place of values as determinants for most behaviours and attitudes. If there is misalignment, then equilibrium is disturbed, and available energy is released chaotically and then the veil of fatigue descends.

My fascination with ART was multi-layered and I was more than intrigued with the way Kaplan as a scholar presented an array of concepts and their connections. It was time to explore how Kaplan's work could be applied to people with

illness-related fatigue, such as cancer, and revitalise the shared interest with
Cimprich (Cimprich 1992, 1993). Three research studies flowed directly out of this
inspiration:

1. *Making the Most Out of Life* (Kirshbaum and Donbavand 2014)
2. *Reiki Experiences in Women Who have Cancer* (Kirshbaum et al. 2016)
3. *Art and ART in Cancer Care* (Kirshbaum et al. 2017; Ennis et al. 2017, 2019)

8.3   Making the Most Out of Life

8.3.1   Background

'Making the most out of life: Exploring the contribution of Attention Restorative
Theory in developing a non-pharmacological intervention for fatigue' (Kirshbaum
and Donbavand 2014) was my first exploratory study inspired and based on
ART. This followed previous studies about cancer-related fatigue, where the emphasis was on encouraging people who have cancer to exercise moderately to improve
their fatigue and overall well-being. However, it was evident that for some individuals, this level of physical exercise is contraindicated and not advised nor desired.
Many people are limited by respiratory, cardiac, neurological or advanced cancer
conditions. Others are restricted by their mobility, flexibility or muscle strength and
will require special considerations or modifications to most exercise prescriptions.
Finally, 'lest we forget', there is also a percentage of the general public who are
blatantly averse to exercise and physical activity although they have been told and
may even accept that it would be beneficial to their health. They will be well versed
in their reasons for being sedentary and might even admit that they are 'excuses',
but their behaviour is determined by individual perception and attitude. To be fair,
physical exercise is not always enjoyable, can be painful and injurious or for some,
the mere thought of movement is torturous and may even trigger unpleasant memories. [My husband tells about his school days in England where cross-country running was something they did when the weather was too harsh for football—they had
to run in the bitter cold rain in shorts.] Nevertheless, I was very interested in determining which other modes of intervention could be suggested for this substantial
group of sufferers of fatigue, aside from the administration of pharmaceutical
agents, which did not seem to be too effective.

8.3.2   Design and Methods

Making the Most Out of Life was planned deliberately to have an upbeat pitch that
was realistic and inclusive of all people who reported having moderate to severe
fatigue, regardless of their diagnosis. In an attempt to be an ethical and considerate
nurse researcher, a positive and uplifting approach was integrated into the design
and research methods in an attempt to minimise directed attention fatigue rather
than rapidly deplete the already limited energy stores of participants any further.

The aim of the study was to determine if ART (Attention Restoration Theory) could be used to develop an effective non-pharmacological intervention to reduce fatigue. The specific research objectives to be achieved at the end of the study were:

1. To identify activities perceived as being enjoyable by individuals who have moderate to severe fatigue related to advanced illness.
2. To determine core attributes of potentially beneficial interventions.
3. To analyse reported 'enjoyable' experiences within the ART framework by mapping emergent themes to the attributes of *attention restoration.*
4. To develop a prototype for a self-management intervention tool for fatigue.

The exploratory, qualitative study guided by the principles of grounded theory took place across three locations: a day hospice, a service user group within the National Health Service (NHS) in the United Kingdom and a podiatry clinic based at the local university where many people had chronic illnesses that caused them to report fatigue as a disturbing, debilitating problem. Prospective participants were screened for inclusion as having at least a moderate level of fatigue using the Edmonton Symptom Assessment System (ESAS) (Bruera et al. 1991), a validated quality of life instrument used in palliative care. Using this scale, a score of 4–10 was required in addition to having a long-term illness or cancer, living at home, and having the ability and desire to participate in a research interview lasting up to 1 h. Anyone who had an acute mental illness or was under 18 years old was excluded from participating.

Following approval from a university-based ethics committee and the research governance group at the hospice, written informed consent was obtained from all participants for open-ended, face-to-face interviews that took place in one of the three locations. Instead of dwelling on the limitations of the participants' current circumstances, the interviews focused on identifying, describing and exploring the qualities of their enjoyable activities or pursuits. In a quiet, comfortable and safe room, contributors were asked simply: 'What do you enjoy doing?' and 'What is it about the activity that you particularly enjoy?' Detailed narratives about each activity such as where, when and how (i.e. alone or with company) were sought to encourage full discovery and exploration of the qualities and characteristics linked to what was perceived as being enjoyable to them. Participants were told that the interview could be stopped at any time, for whatever reason; they just needed to ask. Most of the interviews lasted around 45 min; they were digitally audio-recorded, transcribed, and then analysed using Framework Analysis (Richie and Spencer 1994; Braun and Clark 2006).

Multiple tables were used to record and analyse the text from the transcripts (Miles and Huberman 1994). First, I highlighted all of the identified 'enjoyable activities' for each participant. Then, I transferred the examples to a chart that included additional columns for verbatim quotations and preliminary conceptual or thematic observations, as I began to tease out possible attributes of attention restoration for this population. A full listing of enjoyable activities was generated and then reduced with the input of the rest of the multidisciplinary research team that consisted of academic colleagues from nursing, occupational therapy, physiotherapy and psychology. Members of the research governance group from the local hospice also contributed to streamlining identified enjoyable activities.

8.3.3 Findings

Twenty-five participants were interviewed across the three sites. Just more than half (52%) of the sample had been diagnosed with cancer—the other participants had a broad range of chronic illnesses including chronic obstructive pulmonary disease (COPD), chronic heart disease, end-stage cardiac failure, chronic bronchitis, rheumatoid arthritis, fibromyalgia and diabetes. Sixteen people identified as women and nine as men.

In total, 75 examples of enjoyable activities were identified, described and reflected upon with the objective of exposing latent conceptual themes. Four initial themes emerged from this original study that represented qualities or attributes of energy restorative activities: '*Belonging* (socially engaging), *Expansive* (opportunities for creativity and learning), *Nurturing* (comforting and relaxing) and *Purposeful* (linked to achievement)' (Kirshbaum and Donbavand 2014).

The original article presents each attribute along with participant quotes. Here, I would like to reveal the earliest view of proposed Attributes of Energy Restoration Activities derived from this unique cohort of individuals according to this first study.

8.3.4 The Proposed Attributes of Energy Restoration Activities

From the interviews in the *Making the Most Out of Life* study, *Belonging* was expressed as a social quality, rather than geographical or political, which will be discussed in more detail in Chap. 9. Here, 'the sense of belonging and being a part of the greater community highlighted the value of social engagement and seemed to underlie some of the pleasurable experiences expressed by many participants. This was evident in descriptions of watching and coaching a football match, going out for a meal, dressing up to go to the theatre and interacting with neighbours' (Kirshbaum and Donbavand 2014).

Expansive was associated with taking part in something that extended an individual's daily realm. 'Instead of being bored or frustrated by the limitations of fatigue, there was a substantial subgroup that thrived through seeking out new quests or going forth to learn and develop new talents or abilities. Often it was expressed as the joy of being exposed to something new, different and fascinating such as singing in a choir, going to the theatre, looking at clouds, drawing, learning from books and participating in formal education. One woman in her mothering role described with a bit of a sly smile that she took great pleasure in learning the art of making (and eating) designer cupcakes with her daughter' (Kirshbaum and Donbavand 2014).

Purposeful was an unexpected finding. Enjoyment has many facets and perspectives. What emerged here were numerous accounts of feeling great through taking purposeful action, mainly represented by the mention of involvement in voluntary work and going out of one's way to do something useful. Although participants were living with a chronic or life-threatening illness and were experiencing quite a bit of fatigue, they revealed that they enjoyed and felt it was important to be involved in purposeful acts such as visiting the sick or elderly or starting a support group for people who had rheumatoid arthritis. There was also plenty to be said about compiling a list of tasks and attending to each entry—oh, the joy that comes from the satisfaction of ticking off items on a list, particularly those that have been avoided for months.

Nurturing and nourishing types of activities were also identified. 'In contrast to the individuals that took great pleasure in tackling new challenges, many participants preferred to spend their time in more solitary and comforting ways' (Kirshbaum and Donbavand 2014). The delights of reading, listening to music, being wrapped in warm towels while having a facial in luxurious surroundings and escapist relaxation were well represented.

8.3.5   Discussion

'This study aimed to determine if Attention Restorative Theory (ART), established to improve general wellbeing, could be clinically relevant to the management of illness related fatigue. The intention was to approach the multidimensional, complex, common and persistently distressing symptom from a positive platform, where the emphasis would be upon engaging a person's interest and personal preferences in relation to daytime behaviours. In framing the interviews with the question 'Which activities do you *enjoy*?' participants were led towards describing an array of pleasurable experiences, which was usually an agreeable and cheerful experience for them. However, several people struggled with expressing recent gratifying accounts and were saddened by the realisation that they could only explore enjoyment in terms of referring to their distant past before illness took its toll on their physical and mental health. These disheartening interviews, although few, were upsetting for the novice researchers who, upon de-briefing mentioned that they had asked the question in the past tense e.g. which activities *did* you enjoy? This would have led the participant to place themselves in the past and reflect upon how their health and functional abilities have changed.'

'After many months of continued analysis of the transcripts and consultation within the research team, four overarching attributes of enjoyable activities for this sample were proposed: *Belonging, Expansive, Nurturing* and *Purposeful*. When mapped against the attributes of restorative activities specified in ART (Kaplan 1995), there was some congruence and variation. It was clear that the participants expressed a great need to feel safe and be in a nurturing environment. Some participants placed a high value in and received great joy from contributing to the community; this was not noted in previous ART literature.'

'*Belonging* encapsulates the value of sharing and contributing to the community but also feeling a part of a social gathering such as being with one's family or as part of a theatre audience. Kaplan's *Extent* is most relevant here because it emphases that engagement with an external event or activity is determined by its scope and coherence. There was an aspect of 'normalising' and 'balancing' in relation to social coherence.'

'The attribute of *Expansive* cuts across *Being away, Extent, Compatibility and Fascination* because it is grounded in discovering a particular pursuit that is unique to the individual. It is largely fascinating because it is directly compatible with and dependent upon a person's interests *(Extent)* and provides opportunities for learning and creativity, which take a person away from the mundane and into a new and different place.'

'The attribute of Nurturing in this study resonated most closely with Kaplan's notion of *Being away*, as observed in pleasurable accounts of relaxation, Reiki therapy and being wrapped up warmly. A certain vulnerability and need for security, safety, compassion and care was observed through the participants' words and demeanours. In addition to accrediting restored attention to something that is effortlessly fascinating or eye-catchingly beautiful, respondents in this study frequently stated their commitment and desire to engage with something that had a purpose. It was clear that they took pride in their achievements and efforts, even if it meant that they would need to rest completely for a day or two afterwards to recuperate. In terms of Kaplan's terminology, *Compatibility* and *Extent* appear to be most relevant in terms of the perceptions of purpose. The attribute of *Purposeful* appears to overlap with the themes of *Expansive* and *Belonging* as they relate to the effect and impact of the activity.'

'This study has extended Kaplan's insightful work on restorative behaviours by revealing the value that purposeful, engaging and safe activities hold for people who live with fatigue as a result of advanced cancer or a long-term illness. Furthermore, we conclude that ART has inspired the research team to develop a self-management intervention tool to guide health care practitioners in promoting a non-pharmacological approach to manage fatigue. The prototype of the tool comprises a short interview, an analysis of activities and a co-planning section. Following on from the findings of this study, it is intended to be used to address illness related fatigue through exploring, discovering and promoting experiences which engage, excite, nurture and challenge the person. Further research is needed to advance this approach to strengthen the evidence-base so that a beneficial intervention can be integrated into clinical practice.'

Excerpts from Making the Most Out of Life: Exploring the Contribution of Attention Restorative Theory in Developing a Non-Pharmacological Intervention for Fatigue by Kirshbaum and Donbavand (2014) Palliative and Supportive Care 12(6):473–480: Copyright permission granted from Cambridge University Press 3 March 2021]

8.4   Reiki Experiences in Women Who Have Cancer

8.4.1   Background

The journey to discover interventions, treatment strategies and non-pharmacological approaches to address the widespread symptom of fatigue continued with a small but significant investigation that also attempted to consider the contributions of ART. Following on from all the intensive research I had completed on exercise as an effective intervention for cancer-related fatigue, I felt it was very necessary to address the needs of individuals who were unable to follow the best practice of doing moderate, physical aerobic exercise. Aside from medical interventions that were determined to be considerably limited, what was the alternative for those who had co-morbid, existing or palliative care conditions that were contraindicated to the recommended level and type of physical activity? Although not explicitly directed at cancer-related fatigue, this next study continued to explore well-being and energy restoration within cancer care. However, there was a little twist. Here, a small sample of 10 women diagnosed with cancer were selected to capture their perceptions of their recent experiences of receiving reiki. Could participants in this study of reiki provide some evidence of benefit that linked to ART's attributes of restorative experiences?

Reiki is similar to Therapeutic Touch (Kreiger 1979; Sayre-Adams and Wright 1995) an Energy Therapy, which shares a similar worldview and harmonizes well with Rogers' Science of Unitary Human Beings (please see Chap. 2). The therapeutic approach recognises the permeability of the dynamic energy field that surrounds the person. There is a premise that infinite healing energy is available to anyone who is trained to call it in and able with training to allow it to flow through the body, often through the hands of the practitioner. Then, the practitioner channels it out to where the healing energy is needed. At the very least, a reiki treatment provides the receiver [the client] with a calm, relaxing and holistic experience. The common scenario is for the receiver to be lying on a firm but comfortable treatment, message type of table, in a quiet, temperature-controlled serene room. Sometimes, there is music or candles to promote an environment of calm. However, Reiki can be given to a person sitting in a chair, in bed and also distantly, when the receiver and giver are not even in the same room. There is much to write about reiki—it is fascinating, and even more so when one can confidently record the experiences of those who have received the treatment to improve wellbeing during or following a diagnosis of cancer.

With the purpose of continuing to work with advancing ART through developing an Energy Restoration Framework, I felt it would be useful to delve into the perceptions of reiki generally, as well-being and energy restoration are closely entwined. Would we be able to identify any clear empirical benefits? There were very few published articles in the academic press that had investigated the outcomes of reiki, so there was a gap in the research knowledge that required attention. The plan was to prepare for a full-scale intervention study by first doing a small qualitative pilot study to identify the qualities inherent in the experience and to identify evidenced-based outcome variables for use in a larger intervention study. In addition, the reiki study pilot would provide us with an opportunity to pilot the Self-Management Intervention Tool drafted following the *Making the Most Out of Life.*

8.4.2   Design and Methods

Women who had received at least two reiki sessions at one of three local hospices or at a holistic spa were eligible to participate provided they had received cancer treatment and were in the follow-up, rather than in an active treatment phase of the cancer trajectory. A convenience sample was selected with the assistance of person-nel at the four contributing sites. Semi-structured interviews were conducted that followed a pre-prepared guide that included questions about: 'Why they had chosen to have reiki; Their beliefs and expectations about reiki; What they felt or experi-enced during reiki sessions; How they felt after the reiki session and the duration of any effects; Their views of reiki after receiving it; Any emotional, physical or social effects associated with their experiences of reiki' (Kirshbaum et al. 2016, p. 167).

   Full details of the research plan and selected quotations from the interviews are available in the published article (Kirshbaum et al. 2016), and I would urge you to seek it out if you would like to know more than what is presented here.

8.4.3   Findings

A few points were expressed about the effect of receiving reiki, which were particu-larly exciting to hear and capture. In the course of the interviewing, analysis and synthesis activities, it was revealed that participants experienced a release from the burdensome negative energy that they had not been able to do before. They were able to clear their minds of worry about their cancer and feel an inner peace and welcomed relaxation. This was a space where depression appeared to be lifted out of the physical body and replaced with enjoyment and pleasure. The treasured feel-ing of being cared for and emotionally nourished was expressed frequently.

   Physically, participants spoke of the tangible benefits, such as noticeable pain relief, improved sleep, reduced nausea and reduced abdominal bloating, increased appetite and increased energy. There were also cognitive benefits noticeable in experiencing a greater sense of hope, an improved self-confidence and wanting to participate more in social and community activities. All of these perceived benefits provided the researchers with a descriptive account of the reiki experience that also deepened our conceptual understanding surrounding the attributes of energy resto-ration. The themes of *social belonging, expansion, purposeful* and *nourishment* could be loosely supported and expanded.

8.5 Art in Cancer Care: Exploring the Role of Visual Art-Making and Participatory Performance Programs within an Energy Restoration Framework

The next study took place on the other side of the world, down under in Australia, where I moved to be Professor of Nursing in the tropical Top End based in Darwin, Northern Territory. This time I was very fortunate to meet and begin a magical collaboration with a similarly aligned colleague in social work and an arts producer/curator who shared a very keen interest in integrating creative expression and art-making for people who have undergone cancer treatment. They were also very inter ested in helping me advance the framework that I was developing. In our university-funded research, we organised, facilitated, joined, recorded and evaluated two art-based interventions (Kirshbaum et al. 2017; Ennis et al. 2017, 2019).

1. Art in cancer-care: Exploring the role of visual art-making programs within an Energy Restoration Framework (published in European Journal of Oncology Nursing)
2. The beneficial attributes of visual art-making in cancer care: An integrative review (published in the European Journal of Cancer Care)
3. The energy-enhancing potential of participatory performance-based arts activities in the care of people with a diagnosis of cancer: an integrative review (published in Arts and Health)

This study launched the Energy Restoration Framework where the previous prototype framework from the Kirshbaum and Donbavand study (2014) was fine-tuned into its current conceptual representation. The Art in Cancer Care project was unique through its experiential, not experimental, design. The emphasis was wholeheartedly on participating in art-based group activities and capturing the expressed views of participants about the experience. The research aim was 'to explore the experience of participation in a visual art-making [and performance-based] program for people during and after cancer treatment in the Northern Territory of Australia, using a framework for energy restoration' (Kirshbaum et al. 2017, p. 72).

Two simultaneous, free and artist-facilitated 8-week programs were set up in local community spaces. The small sample of 16 people was divided into two groups that met either on Tuesday or Wednesday, at two different venues. Each venue was suited to the arts-based activities that took place at weekly intervals in the early evening. Venue 1 was a community arts and craft centre, where visual art-making activities such as still-life painting, papier-mâché pots, fibre sculpture, weaving and natural silk scarf dying were led by two professional local artists.

The venue was a light, airy space with high wooden benches where people could sit or stand to create their artwork. The centre is surrounded by a natural park-like environment by the sea. (Kirshbaum et al. 2017 p. 73)

Venue Two was the dance studio of a local community dance company. The room was an open space and had polished wooden flooring and a fully mirrored wall. The main group-based activities that took place here were in the realm of theatre-craft, which included a wide range of exploratory exercises incorporating drama, singing, movement and dance and visual tableau performance. This group was led by a vibrant and talented drama teacher, actress and theatre producer. We shared many fun and heart-opening moments as we explored our voices, bodies, perceptions, interpretations and trust in others in some pretty crazy and creative ways, sometimes challenging our coordination and concentration skills in the process.

We gathered mainly qualitative information before, during and after the art-making experiences for both the groups. The Interview Guide to Energy Restoration in the Self-Management of Fatigue was used as a basis for a semi-structured interview that took place following informed consent and before the first of the 8-week series of art-making. At this preliminary interview, participants were asked about the kinds of art-based activities they have enjoyed throughout different periods in their life, while delving into their conceptualisations of attributes of the Energy Restoration Framework: *Nurturing, Belonging, Purposeful* and *Expansive*. Also, at this interview, we discussed their preference for attending the visual or performance stream of art-based activities and were allocated to the relevant group according to their preference.

At the start of each session, a brief check-in and review of the past week within each group was led by one of the researchers and audio-recorded. A one-item Likert-type scale of well-being was administered before and also after each session which used 'smiley faces' ranging from very happy to very sad, with an invitation to record a few words about how they feel. This allowed the research team to capture the potential effect of the intervention by analysing the potential change in mood and general emotional state of participants.

The final individual in-depth interview took place at the end of the art-making program. Here, the focus was on the participants' descriptions and deeper perceptions of their recent experiences. Analysis of the interview transcripts followed Template Analysis that began with a priori themes, which were the attributes of the Energy Restorative Framework (Kirshbaum and Donbavand 2014); these were refined through integrating, interpreting, reflecting upon and confirming findings (King 1998; Crabtree and Miller 1999; Brooks et al. 2015). NVIVO software was used as a tool to record and categorise the qualitative data from all sources.

The original four a priori themes were retained and a fifth was identified as *Stimulating*. In addition, subthemes emerged which served to deepen and broaden conceptualisation of the Framework as demonstrated in Table 8.1:

The art-based program was a valued and beneficial experience for participants, facilitator/artists and the research team. The previously identified attributes were extended and confirmed. Specifically, the theme of expansion was highly regarded so much so that an additional theme of *stimulation* provided excitement that provided intrigue and positive anticipation prior to each session. We were able to obtain sufficient evidence of uplifting and energising effects that lasted into the next subsequent week. There was an observable improvement in mood and sense

Table 8.1 Attributes of energy restoration in cancer and palliative care context (Kirshbaum et al. 2017, p. 74)

Theme/Attribute	Subtheme
Expansive	Development of self
	Intention to continue
	Learning a skill/gaining knowledge
Belonging	Effect of the group
	Observing the group
	Sharing the fun
Nurturing	People
	Relaxing, not stressful
	Safe to create
Purposeful	Achievement
	Commitment
Stimulating	Anticipation
	Duration of effect
	Environment
	Fascinating/absorbing
	Uplifting and energising

Reprinted with permission from Elsevier from European Journal of Oncology Nursing

of freedom that accompanied the art-based sessions, which was expressed by one participant as:

> It's been exhilarating and very, very helpful to me to get out and to do something (Kirshbaum et al. 2017, p. 76).

The sense of *Belonging* was also extremely noteworthy. The presence and exuberance of the facilitator/artists were evidenced by their openness, enthusiasm, uniqueness and encouragement. These qualities were interpreted as fostering creativity, increased well-being through the significant immersion into art-based activities and the experience of welcomed expansion through creative flow. These results were truly heart-warming for all involved.

The adaption of Kaplan's Attention Restoration Theory (ART) to cancer and palliative populations became a reality through the exploratory qualitative studies presented in this chapter. The attributes that had previously been identified to explain why some actions used to restore attention in an involuntary way, such as: *extent, being away, compatibility, fascination,* had now been altered to reflect the experiences of illness-specific cohorts. I had not intended to refute Kaplan's work but rather investigate ART under different conditions, where fatigue was attributed to the multidimensional domains of a physical illness.

The resultant attributes/themes and their sub-themes from the research are subjective at this stage. Continued knowledge building is required to expand and deepen the conceptual understanding of each attribute through concept analyses and a series of individual systematic reviews across associated disciplines that includes nascent scientific advances. Aside from keeping me happily occupied and cognitively nourished and expanded, I am convinced that these two major research-based enhancements will enable me to improve the specificity and coherence of the developing framework.

In the next chapter I will present the emergent Energy Restoration Framework and begin to explain how it could be used in practice.

References

Braun V, Clark V. Using thematic analysis in psychology. Qual Res Psychol. 2006;3:77–101.

Brooks J, McCluskey S, Turley E, King. The utility of template analysis in qualitative psychology research. Qual Res Psychol. 2015;12(2):202–22.

Bruera E, Kuehn N, Miller MJ, Selmser P, Macmillan K. The Edmonton symptom assessment system (ESAS): a simple method for the assessment of palliative care patients. J Palliat Care. 1991;7:6–9.

Cimprich B. Attentional fatigue following breast cancer surgery. Res Nurs Health. 1992;15:199–207.

Cimprich B. Development of an intervention to restore attention in cancer patients. Nurs Res. 1993;16:83–92.

Crabtree BF, Miller WL, editors. Doing qualitative research. Quebec: Sage; 1999.

Ennis G, Kirshbaum MN, Waheed N. The beneficial attributes of visual art- making in cancer care: an integrative review. Eur J Cancer Care. 2017;29:71–8. https://doi.org/10.1111/ecc.12663.

Ennis G, Kirshbaum M, Waheed N. The energy-enhancing potential of participatory performance-based arts activities in the care of people with a diagnosis of cancer: an integrative review. Arts Health. 2019;11(2):87–103. https://doi.org/10.1080/17533015.2018.1443951.

James W. Psychology. The briefer course. New York: Holt; 1892.

Kaplan S. The restorative benefits of nature: toward an integrative framework. J Environ Psychol. 1995;15:169–82.

Kaplan S. Meditation, restoration and the management of mental fatigue. Environ Behav. 2001;33:480–506.

Kaplan R, Basu A. Fostering reasonableness: supportive environments for bringing out the best. Michigan: Maize Books; 2015.

Kaplan S, Kaplan R, editors. Humanscape: environments for people. Duxbury: Belmont, CA; 1978. (Republished by Ann Arbor, MI: Ulrich's, 1982.)

Kaplan S, Kaplan R. Cognition and environment: functioning in an uncertain world. New York: Praeger; 1982.

King N. Template analysis. In: Symon G, Cassell C, editors. Qualitative methods and analysis in Organiazational research. London: Sage; 1998.

Kirshbaum M, Donbavand J. Making the most out of life: exploring the contribution of attention restorative theory in developing a non-pharmacological intervention for fatigue. Palliat Support Care. 2014;12(6):473–80.

Kirshbaum M, Olson K, Pongthavornkamol K, Graffigna. Understanding the meaning of fatigue at the end of life: an ethnoscience study. Eur J Oncol Nurs. 2012;17:146–53. https://doi.org/10.1016/j.ejon.2012.04.007.

Kirshbaum MN, Stead M, Bartys. An exploratory study of reiki experiences in women who have cancer. Int J Palliat Nurs. 2016;22(4):166–72.

Kirshbaum M, Ennis G, Waheed N. Art in cancer care: exploring the role of visual art-making programs within an energy restoration framework. Eur J Oncol Nurs. 2017;29:71–8. https://doi.org/10.1016/j.ejon.2017.05.003.

Kreiger D. The therapeutic touch: how to use your hands to help or heal. New York: Prentice Hall; 1979.

Miles MB, Huberman AM. Qualitative data analysis. 2nd ed. Thousand Oaks: Sage; 1994.

National Comprehensive Cancer Network (NCCN). Cancer-related fatigue: NCCN clinical practice guidelines in oncology; 2020. https://www.nccn.org/professionals/physician_gls/pdf/fatigue.pdf

Richie J, Spencer L. Qualitative data analysis for applied policy research. In: Bryman A, Burgess RG, editors. Analyzing qualitative data. London: Routeledge; 1994.

Sayre-Adams, Wright. The theory and practice of therapeutic touch. Edinburgh: Churchill Livingstone; 1995.

Sullivan W. In search of a clear head. In: Kaplan R, Basu A, editors. Fostering reasonableness: supportive environments for bringing out the best. Michigan: Maize Books; 2015.

9.1 Introduction

From my research thus far, which includes many years of experiential immersion (Fig. 9.1), five core attributes of restorative expression have been postulated, tested, revised, applied and amended for the purpose of driving forward a vision for a health and wellness program called the Joyful Freedom Approach. I will discuss this in the next chapter. Now I will take some time and space to present the foundation to the Joyful Freedom Approach, which is the Energy Restoration Framework. Here in this chapter, you will find the definitions of key terms, assumptions, attributes and the summarised framework (Table 9.1).

The five attributes are conceptual in their development, scope and application to energy creation and sustenance. Currently, I am referring to them using the acronym PECAN: **P**urposeful, **E**xpansive, **C**onnecting/Belonging, **A**we-Inspiring and **N**ourishing, although as I will explain, they are not completely static just yet. Each attribute represents infinite types and qualities of activities or pursuits [Expressions according to the Framework] that can be explored, reviewed and then integrated into an individual daily or weekly routine. This process relies on the person being open to reflecting and instigating small changes that could reap large benefits by creating energy and being freed from debilitating fatigue and lethargy. Some would say it encourages delving deep into one's heart-space or into their soul to entice an individual's innate joy to emerge. Reconnecting with joy, in its broadest interpretation, is a central part of addressing fatigue. Concurrently, the framework acknowledges the importance of bringing awareness to the blocks and barriers that limit the full positive, joyful expression of a person's emotional, spiritual, sexual, functional, social, physical and cognitive self.

The Framework uses the attributes conceptually as they represent more than just a word or term, but each can be explored from different perspectives and studied deeply; each will lead to creative modes and programs for *lifelong optimal self-care*.

© Springer Nature Switzerland AG 2021   111
M. N. Kirshbaum, *The Joyful Freedom Approach to Cancer-Related Fatigue*,
https://doi.org/10.1007/978-3-030-76932-1_9

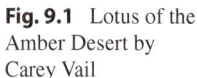

Fig. 9.1 Lotus of the
Amber Desert by
Carey Vail

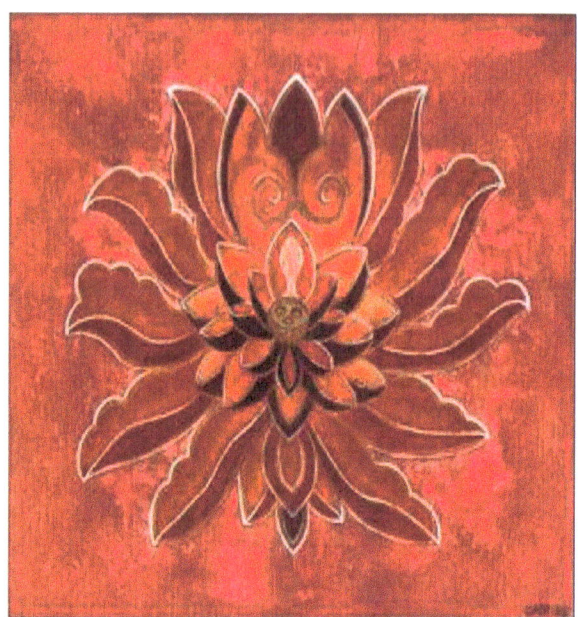

The framework is intended to be used flexibly and be adapted as needed for diverse populations, in addition to those who live with cancer-related fatigue.

I have been using my own recent experience of recovery from open-heart surgery to critique and refine what I have postulated and piloted through empirical research. Although I have not had cancer, recovery from major surgery entails a fair amount of illness-related fatigue to deal with and its fair share of emotional and physical pain.

Cancer-related fatigue (CRF) has many direct and indirect causes, many occurring concurrently. The Joyful Freedom Approach and the Energy Restoration Framework that underpins the program will not be able to 'cure' anyone of fatigue—it is not a magic bullet or 'pill'. It merely attempts to gently guide the person towards discovering practical ways to create and use beneficial energy that abounds. I view this as a *lifelong self-care* priority that can be applicable to everybody—not only for those who have experienced CRF but also their family, friends, healthcare practitioners and anyone else who feels they could benefit from this type of approach.

After much deliberation, I have decided to classify the Energy Restoration Framework as an integrative framework, as it is intended to encourage exploratory and experimental momentum. The Framework is inherently action-based and relies on the client/patient doing some 'inner work' on themselves, guided by a counsellor or other healthcare professional to assist them to make creative adjustments to their lives. Each of the five identified attributes acts as a self-analysis prompt from where enlivening and energy-management interventions can be identified, initiated,

Table 9.1 The Energy Restoration Framework: attributes, elements, domains and expressions

Attributes (PECAN)	Elements [the what] (dominant domains)	Expressions [the how] (Examples of pursuits and activities to be explored shamelessly and without reserve)
P–purposeful	Planning and completing tasks (functional, physical)	Washing the kitchen floor, sewing on a button
	Planning and completing achievements (cognitive, physical)	Studying for an academic degree, running a marathon
	Community service and political activism (social, political)	Volunteering at a food bank, organising a rally against racism
	Initiating movement (physical)	Taking a brisk walk to greet the sunrise every morning
E–expansive	Learning and developing skills (cognitive)	Learning a foreign language
	Venturing into a new role (functional)	Identifying as an artist and making art
	New view of self (emotional)	Taking the challenge and leading an event
	New environment (physical)	Travel and engaging with new situations, sights and people
C–connecting	Experiencing shared values (functional, spiritual, political)	Joining a meditation group or amateur dance troupe
	Participating in shared activities (social)	Planning an event with others
	Ease/effortless state (emotional)	Catching up with a dear friend and talking about anything and everything that comes to mind
A–awe inspiring	Observing nature (physical)	Watching a seed pop through the soil or the patterns that tiny crabs make on the sand
	Anticipation (emotional)	Excited and so happy about learning the next dance routine
	Mesmerising (spiritual, cognitive)	Watching the moon and aura emerge from the lattice of clouds and then observe their disappearance
N–nourishing	Nurturing the six senses (physical, spiritual) Sight, sound, touch, taste, smell, intuition	Walking on the beach in the tropics, feeling pleasure
	Comfort (physical, emotional)	A warm, fragrant bath; a delightful meal full of colour and healthy goodness
	Cultivating the intellect (cognitive)	Listening to a master storyteller

integrated and revised. The Framework provides a structure that can be used by the individual and practitioner together as they co-develop a dynamic action plan that can be reviewed and revised at regular intervals as needed.

At some point, most of us will be hampered by feelings of being stuck in a rut. This might be accompanied by hopelessness, frustration, anger or despair. The suggested approach encourages us all to break out of previous detrimental patterns and routines and commit to shaking things up a bit—to take on more of a pioneering approach—to go forth on a new path, without any preconceived limits. The onus is on the person, with guidance and support from a healthcare professional or alternative, holistic practitioner to develop expertise in sculpting a practical approach to stimulating the production of useable energy and promoting an easy flow to where it is needed most.

It is postulated that these attributes and the simple structure provided by the Framework may hold the keys to living a joyful, healthy and vibrant life, particularly after destabilising, disruptive, debilitating and energy-draining life events.

9.2   Definitions

Energy refers to the vast array of forces behind all forms of movement and reactivity. Utilization of the framework is intended to increase the availability of enlivening, creative and motivational energies that are, in essence, therapeutic and healing as opposed to being destructive and harmful.

Restoration in this context refers to the restoration of vitality and wellbeing to the person. *Restoration* has been used because the framework was inspired directly from Kaplan's Attention Restorative Theory (Chap. 8) and adapted following a series of small research studies in the United Kingdom and Australia. *Energy* replaced *Attention* to signify the major shift in emphasis from academics and then the general population associated with the way information was received within the field of environmental psychology, to people who were experiencing illness-related fatigue. In contrast to being concerned with the tiredness that results from *directed attention,* which we all experience when we are in situations that require us to focus intently on an activity and shut out the external environment, the framework aims to assist people who have depleted their stored energy due to a disruptive circumstance, such as illness, medical-surgical treatment or distressing life events. Still, in this context, the aim has always been to restore energy to the person. To do this, usable energy needs to be created to enable it to flow to where it is needed most and to fortify the person as they face the many challenges inherent in an unwanted or inevitable disruptive experience.

Lifelong self-care emphasizes that all that we do or try to do regularly to promote good health should be viewed as ongoing. Self-care gets mentioned quite a bit these days as people realise the value of taking responsibility for their own health and become less reliant upon medical practitioners, particularly in terms of the prevention of illness, reducing harmful stress and generally seeking health-related information to improve well-being and minor, non-critical or life-threatening events.

9.3   Assumptions

All life is dynamic and in a state of ongoing change. From the miraculous moments of conception and then birth, we are immersed in our space-time, where we grow, develop, learn and age.

We are sensual and sensitive beings who are constantly adjusting to the ever-changing internal and external energies that surround us.

By making subtle alterations in our perceptions and actions, we can calm, balance and energise our mood state. The way this is done, and our available resources, will vary according to every unique individual. This should be accepted, honoured and celebrated, along with our inherent diversity.

We exist in multiple dimensions, simultaneously.

Although the majority of us can only envision and comprehend our most dominant world through our six senses: sight, smell, touch, hearing, taste and intuition, our perceptions are not rigid or fixed. Small shifts in observation, experiences and consciousness can shift mood, be stimulating and therefore increase feelings of vitality and vigour. Each of our senses can be augmented through practice and exercises as evidenced in the wonderful diversity of Indigenous, ethnic, religious and cultural traditions across the globe who recognize the presence of spirits, celestial beings, animal guides, ancestors and descents who have not been born to this world yet.

9.4   Overview of the Framework

The Energy Restoration Framework (Table 9.1) is presented here in a simple table across three columns that sets out the core, proposed structure. The first column lists the five attributes, which will be described in turn below, according to the acronym PECAN. PECAN does not have any particular symbolism, aside from memories of American hot pecan pie with ice cream; it just makes the attributes easy to remember and use when checking-in with oneself and as a self-assessment feature within the program for *lifelong self-care*. The second column identifies elements and their most dominant domains as branches or subthemes relative to the five attributes. The elements and domains are intended to help an individual look within themselves to become more acutely aware of what motivates and soothes them and also to look outside themselves and explore other ways of being *purposeful, expansive, connecting, awe-inspiring or nourishing* [the attributes]. Then, the experimentation with different expressions of the elements can begin. Column three of the Framework provides some example expressions. I propose that for each element, a list is drawn up of possible pursuits or activities that can be explored if desired. These examples of expressions can then be reviewed and analysed simply, and if energizing and enjoyable, added to an on-going, unbounded, lifelong listing that can serve as a reference guide/toolkit for when energy is depleted and in need of a boost! The elements, their dominant domains and expressions are intended to remind the person of what has previously worked well for them in terms of changing from low energy to a higher energy, vitalized state.

9.5   Attributes

9.5.1   Purposeful

Consider living every day of your life without a defined purpose. Is it even possible, I wonder? Yes, it would be fabulous to be a total free-spirit and just do whatever you desired without guilt. This is so valued when I am on vacation and am able to plan to not have a plan for each and every moment of the usual merry-go-round of work, home, family, exercise, classes/courses, socialising and so on. But I know that I get a massive burst of energy in the form of excitement when I complete something—anything. It could be as basic as ticking items off on a to do list of errands, through to the very emotional personal achievement of finally being awarded a PhD following many years of adversity.

For the attribute of *Purposeful,* four elements and dominant domains were identified as:

Planning and completing personal tasks (functional, physical)
Planning and completing life achievements (cognitive, physical)
Community service and political activism (social, political)
Initiating movement (physical)

The Oxford Dictionary defines purpose in two ways: (1) the reason for which something is done or created or for which something exists and (2) a person's sense of resolve or determination. Both descriptions provide a core functional and foundational element to why an individual would move forward in a focused and determined way. The person is driven to do something with a clear purpose, rather than cruise around waiting to respond. Without diversion or distraction, the defined purpose has a chance of being achieved, whatever its size or level of importance.

I came across a very interesting book by Brian A Garner called Garner's Modern English Usage (Garner 2016) in which the author clarifies different usages of words and their roots. Under *purposeful* he writes, 'see *purposive,*' which to me makes me think of purposive sampling, done mainly within qualitative research studies. Garner presents the differences between *purposely = on purpose, intentionally* and *purposefully = with a specific purpose in mind.* For *purposeful,* he draws on the Oxford dual meaning: (1) having a purpose and (2) full of determination.

When looking at the meaning of words, I always find it useful to look to other disciplines. I came across Wilson's *Designing the Purposeful Organisation* (Wilson 2015) where the author approaches the concept of purpose through the lens of organisational management. Here the words of *purpose* and *purposeful* are huge drivers to the success of the collective and the individual within the organisation. For example, Wilson writes that purpose is:

> the [strategic] anchor for all we do and that performance is dependent on harmonisation and synergising our purpose … crafting our purpose is at the core of inspiring business to perform beyond boundaries …

Purpose tells us why we're here and vision tells us where we're going … Our vision identi-
fies what is important and gives clues to the structures we should put in place for efficient
delivery.

Early on Wilson presents a formula that identifies three components to results and success:

Alignment = Strength and Focus = Energy focused consistently = Results and success.

This is the high end of why identifying and following through with a purpose are important. My interpretation is that there needs to be coherence between the components to achieve desired outcomes. I believe this would be valuable for us all to remember. Ideally, when someone has a clearly defined purpose, there is a force to grow, create and thrive. However, once someone is thrown off balance, there is a likelihood that they will struggle and fall prey to unintended or undesirable circumstances unless they are able to return once again to their purpose, realign themselves to it and take determined action. And this is one excellent way to get motivated, invigorated and energised and begin to create more energy from within oneself. I was inspired by Wilson's book because it has an energising flow—the intention and determination of the author to deliver on his *purpose* shine through. It looks like it would be very useful to all leaders and managers too, by the way.

Purposeful is different from meaningful, which is existential and could be seen as relating to the meaning of life. This can be argued—but not here. When someone is trying their best to feel well, do what they enjoy and attend to the multitude of responsibilities they think are so important, but gets struck down by the familiar and distressing symptom that defines their fatigue, then identifying a purposeful activity or task can be surprisingly effective. Even getting up out of bed, having a shower, getting dressed, eating breakfast, brushing teeth, settling down with a good book or taking a little nap can be very satisfying if framed as a purposeful triumph and a 'why not?' attitude. Furthermore, creative and concrete projects that start with a vision and then get completed such as an acrylic painting on a large canvas or varnishing a garden fence can also be energising. Purposeful is contextual—it depends on the person and their desires, skills and abilities within a particular environment and for a particular function.

The drive to complete a planned single task can be strengthened when an individual realises that the value of the task extends beyond the observable accomplishment and will provide motivation and enthusiasm for the rest of the day. The very act of completing something creates energy in itself. It is a very subtle way to move out of debilitating lethargy and even despair.

It may be difficult for the person who has a scattered mind and struggles to make a decision, any decision, even a very small one. We need to understand that and be aware and sensitive to the 'monkey mind' that is unsettled and restless, as it is also a contributor to fatigue as an energy zapper. In this situation, a written list that is dynamic and ongoing is recommended. Examples of tasks that might have been floating around the mind for eons can be jotted down in a specific notebook or file and then the person [with the scattered mind] is instructed to just chose one to address, knowing that there is no preference—all tasks have equal value here. It is the beginning to move, generate and shift available energy that is important.

9.5.2   Expanding/Expansive

The bountiful attribute of *expanding* was birthed from the consciousness of people who were actively living with a diagnosis of cancer. The joy of extending beyond one's usual boundaries through learning or doing something new was observed and expressed in several early studies. However, it was within the container of the small, relatively recent experiential research study, where the quality of expansion and role in creating usable energy was recounted most profoundly. This Australian-based project (Ennis et al. 2017, 2019, Kirshbaum et al. 2017) set out to capture the impact of facilitated art-making within a group and in doing so, revealed something quite potent and unexpected. It turns out that having opportunities for all kinds of expansive experiences is tremendously valued. It might be because expansion provides an optimistic, hopeful and forward-gazing lens that links the present to the future, but I am just speculating here.

It is hard waking up in the morning knowing that your day might be dominated by the effects of your illness. You might have lived with an illness for a long time and have internalised the role of the 'sick person' for longer than you would have liked. Yet, you plod on and face the day, doing your best to overcome some of the routine challenges and acute complications as they arise. Now, what about spending an evening gathering some roots, seeds and flowers in a tropical location and learning how to tie-dye a silk scarf using natural resources? Which roots are best? How do I get a blue colour? What else can I add in? How should I tie it to get that beautiful crinkly effect? Am I mixing it correctly in the brewing cauldron? Oh, this is fun … I can't wait to see what my scarf will look like when it is finished! Oh, how stunning!! And I did it!

The experience of just doing something new, in a safe group, was energising for the participants in this art-making study—and the effect continued as folks could draw on the memory and relive their excitement. Instead of talking about their cancer journeys, which they could if they wanted to, conversation within the art room was about their art-making. The artifacts: songs sheets, photos of tableaus, poems, jewellery, paintings, sculptures and papier mâché pots infused memories that were available to enliven the participants long after they were created.

This project was very pleasing to do, but what added to the honour was hearing about the expansive effects from the participants. Not only did the participants enjoy the sessions, but they were able to put aside their aches, pains and worries and become artists. The exposure to 'another world' was uplifting and carried on having an impact on their whole 'view of self', which if viewed through an existential lens, is truly deep.

Social and behaviour scientists provide much discourse around concepts of self-efficacy (Bandura 1977), self-concept (Mattingly and Lewandowski 2013, 2014) and the relationship between these two super concepts as being important determinants of behaviour change, particularly during tough times. Dys-Steenbergen et al.

(2016) and Aron and Aron (1986) demonstrate the relationship between self-efficacy and self-concept in their Self-Expansive Model. This model proposes that a basic motivation exists within the individual that enhances personal efficacy through seeking out new resources, perspectives, and identities; these work to promote the achievement of present and future goals. Mattingly and Lewandowski (2013, 2014) contribute interesting discussions on self and reality concluding that an expanded self is a more capable self.

In our context, learning something in a safe and comfortable group setting gave people confidence not only to make and participate in an art activity but also to go out of the house, socialise and explore a bit. Complementary to the earlier studies, it was found that travel, all kinds of learning and skill development and venturing out into other roles were all indicative of the stimulation and excitement inherent in expansive activities. The resultant elements and dominant domains were narrowed down to: Learning and developing skills (cognitive), Venturing into a new role (functional), New view of self (emotional) and New environment (physical).

The attribute of *Expansive* recognises that a rigid, blocked and shocked human energy field will struggle to exist. Through introducing activities and situations in one's everyday life that gently encourage a change in roles and expectations can help people break out of a rut or the feeling of being stuck. In addition, the quality of *Expanding* deals with the expansion of thought, of boundaries and sometimes requires the person to let go of past behaviours, attitudes, views, perceptions, lenses and filters.

Expansive and Expanding

We expand our views.

We expand our horizons and look beyond what we normally see, or go beyond our previously assumed boundaries. We release limitations, fears, restrictions.

We expand our minds to explore something new—a language, body of knowledge, go beyond what we thought was possible. Here we encourage and promote and become open to challenges. We learn. We welcome in challenge, novelty—it's exciting and invigorating! It is energy creating—can you see it dear readers?

We expand beyond what we thought was possible, what we thought was safe, possible.

We expand our view of ourselves and welcome in creativity and right hemisphere of the brain activity. We can expand the palette of colours or style of our dress or hair.

We can expand and pay more attention to each of our senses including the 6th sense of intuition, and bring in greater depth and complexity, if we so desire.

We can do all this consciously but may benefit from encouraging words or actions to get us started. [i.e. toolkit and action planning of the Joyful Freedom Approach]

9.5.3   Connecting/Belonging

It is not only energy fields that are constantly in flux. The current framework remains a work in progress and is dynamic and adaptive to continued revelations, several of which I have come across in my dreams and then found myself bolt upright and utter to myself—'of course, that makes more sense'. *Belonging* and before that, the linguistically abhorrent, *Belongingness,* were the words that I was using to capture a social and value-based quality. The original phrase, *Social Belonging*, was an early analytical code to depict the yearning that some participants felt to be a part of something. This followed the dissociation and loneliness they experienced through cancer treatment and recovery. One dear woman in an early study told me that she walked around the village each day as a way of feeling connected to where she lived and its people. She did not have to join a group, be considered worthy, or share political values with anyone necessarily, it was just the act of having a wander and saying hello to the locals that perked her up socially. The more extreme extroverts that I interviewed were used to gaining an energy boost through interacting with others. So, for them, the months of reduced socializing were extra tough. Going out and being with friends or social groups provided the much-needed social interaction and lively environment that helped to invigorate them.

Connecting, the current word to identify the attribute, is now considered preferable because it is less aligned to the broader political and social tensions that I came across in the literature on *Belonging. Connecting* feels more earthy and physical to me; it does not involve debates or justifications related to national identity or rights of immigrants and refugees. I am sensitive to these issues because of my past. I am now a citizen of a third country. After being born in the United States, living there for 24 years, and then moving to England for another huge chunk of my history, I am now in the Northern Territory of Australia where I have lived for 7 years. Am I Australian? Do I belong here? These are not easy questions to answer. However, I have many connections here, which enables me to feel relaxed, nourished, loved, intrigued and valued. The more connections I experience and the greater their intensity provides me with feelings of well-being, which I cherish greatly.

Connecting is an attribute of energy restoration because when someone feels like they belong or have a special connection to a place, object, expression of art (dance, music), community or fellow human being, one is more apt to feel at ease and safe. When you are amongst people who accept you unconditionally and can just 'be' with the object of your connection, you can feel freed from the constraints that bind your thoughts, speech and actions. There is less of a need to be on your guard for fear of saying or doing something 'out of line'. If you are connecting to a song, special tree, crystal or cuddly teddy bear, for example, you might feel like you are in a bubble of meditative contentment or 'in the zone' of pleasant concentration or contemplation—and this, my dear readers, provides the space for healing, life force energy to gather and work its magic.

Connecting is an important positively vectored aspect of so much that we do. We are social beings born into a ready-made social network, that is the family. Throughout our lives, we keep joining other social networks such as school, work and leisure pursuits. However, joining a network is not enough to benefit in terms of energy restoration; this is realized once we notice that we share beliefs, values and even wild aspirations and visions with others. Then something extraordinary occurs—we connect—and from there, we can soar.

Belonging is a very personal feeling. Sometimes we yearn to be part of something. Something we may feel while experiencing despair but not know the precise cause. We might come to the conclusion that something is missing in our lives—this very well could be a supportive connection. I would venture to say that we all have memories and experiences of this deep longing. We may be lonely and feel no one cares, or no one shares our interests, or we are in pain or disabled and cut off from others. We may experience inaccessibility and isolation due to where we live, availability of transport, technophobia (when the world seems to expect online communications and virtuosity of the 'smart phone') or a whole range of physical and mental disabilities that often accompany normal ageing that might make connecting and connection difficult.

Some of us have issues of shame, so we do not feel that we will ever belong or make meaningful social connections because of what we have done or thought. The artist, dreamworker and author Toko-Pa Turner has written a mesmerizing book on her personal journey that goes into substantial depth surrounding *Belonging, Remembering Ourselves Home* (Turner 2017). I recommend it highly. There are insights that are integrated with an intelligent and wise perspective. For many of us, we may recognize a desire to be part of 'something', but we do not feel worthy of joining or being truly accepted by others. We might presume we need to be accepted to belong. However, *Belonging*, from a subjective perspective, is in our minds and hearts. When we ask ourselves: 'Do I belong here?', the formulation of the response may trigger a host of discordant beliefs. In the least helpful viewpoint, we place ourselves into a position where we are seeking approval from others, instead of just striding into a room confidently, shining our light, full of charisma, self-esteem and determination. A more enlivened and empowered approach would be to say to yourself, 'I belong here, because I am here, right here. That is the truth, this is where I am now. I should not have to waste my energy contemplating what others think of me.' I offer these words as an oncology nurse, who has counselled so many women with lowered self-esteem following cancer treatment. So much precious effort was wasted trying to be accepted by others, instead of using their limited energy resources to empower their inner 'control centre' and strengthen their energy field.

If we go back to the Framework (Table 9.1), we can see that the attribute of *Connecting/Belonging* has three elements and dominant domains: Experiencing shared values (spiritual, functional, political), Participating in shared activities (social) and Ease/effortless state (emotional). How wonderful would it be to increase our connection experiences and benefit from the feeling of being a part of 'something' that you cherish? As for all the elements listed in the Framework, they are intended to help formulate an individual toolkit of expressions/activities, which can then be tried and tested. So, how can you or your clients/patients address the elements for *Connecting/Belonging*? In which ways can you go forth and find an activity to share, or a person that shares something unique with you? Can you think of a time when you felt the warmth and ease of connection? Bring the memory back into your consciousness—tap into the feeling. Can you feel a spark that enlivens your spirit? Violà! Energy is created.

9.5.4   Awe-Inspiring/Fascinating/Stimulating

Do you ever get bored? Or find yourself in situations that are uninteresting and just taking up your time? You might try to convince yourself that these tasks or circumstances serve some underlying or indirect purpose. Perhaps this chore or responsibility is part of your job so you get on with it, or maybe you convince yourself that you are being respectful or kind to someone else—you wouldn't want to be rude, would you? Or maybe you have been diagnosed with cancer or another illness and have been undergoing medical treatment leaving you feel run-down and low on usable energy?

Whatever the cause of you feeling uninspired, a spark of intrigue is required. I am convinced, having confirmed this so many times with clients and myself, that just a little spark of interest can ignite the fire within you. It is remarkable that it might only take a moment to shift your energy level.

Fascination was an overarching conceptual quality that Stephen Kaplan (Kaplan 1995, 2001) used in his Attention Restoration Theory (ART), rather than an individual attribute. I resisted including it in my research as I analysed the ART in art-making study with my co-researchers. However, it was just too important to the research participants as an attribute of energy restoration. When people talked about participating in the art-making sessions, we witnessed their excitement and joy. The spark of intrigue was ignited and witnessed. When we analysed the interview transcripts, and were left with only the words on the screen, without the twinkle in participants' eyes or the smiles that lit up their faces, the descriptions oozed energy. This is something that we knew we had to keep as a core attribute, although found it hard to decide what to call it: *stimulating* or *fascinating*? I then stumbled on another highly readable and pertinent book called *Phosphorescence: On Awe, Wonder & Things that Sustain You When the World Goes Dark* by Julia Baird (Baird 2020). The words *awe* and *wonder* captured my attention. So, for now, I am calling the attribute *awe-inspiring* and moving on!

We can find wonder and *awe-inspiring* opportunities everywhere; an infinite number if we are able to stop and use our senses. Look closely at anything and you will see patterns. Notice the innate aesthetics and be invited to appreciate the intricate complexity [in other circumstances: wild messy chaos] or pure simplicity that is inherent in all things. Isn't it fascinating that you might never have noticed such detail or beauty before? I would urge you to explore what is around the proverbial corner. Speak, or rather, listen to someone intently with your absolute, full attention. Each time we allow ourselves to pause consciously, a moment that could have been mundane, becomes transformed into something spectacular. I like to call this magic—but it is really down to being open and welcoming to greet the full spectrum and *awe-inspiring* depth of our surroundings.

And then there are more stereotypical examples of magnificent and fascinating sights, people and experiences that are included in the attribute of what I am now calling for now: *awe-inspiring.* Where I live there are many waterfalls whose waters rage in abundance following a prolonged and intense rainy season. Catching a single or double rainbow over the sea or field is spectacular. I am lucky to live on the coast, where the sun, moon and the stars pass on their luminescence over to the water, where the mesmerizing sound of the waves is heard relentlessly throughout the night. I recently sighted a manta-ray playing about in the sea, showing its shark-like fin—but was it a shark? Wow!

From my world, I can share that I find the act of putting paint on paper pretty awesome, particularly when I am open to the creative, easy mode and can move the brush flowingly. I also find fascination in the artwork of professional artists, word-scapes of poets and relish the incredible beauty, athleticism and outrageous synchronic movements of performing dancers. I am sure that you will all be able to list plenty of examples that grab your attention and invoke a sense of wonder that is unique to you and your perceptions. I would encourage you to jot down a few *awe-inspiring* expressions and refer back to the list when you feel a bit energy depleted. Observe the effect of just thinking about one or two expressions. You might find yourself uplifted, just through the action of pondering and reflecting. Well, this is an objective of the Energy Restoration Framework—to explore what provides you and your clients with that special little spark of energy to boost mood and help to address the undesirable aspects of fatigue and lethargy.

9.5.5 Nourishing/Nurturing and Nourishment

This attribute of the Framework emerged from my early research studies of fatigue in cancer and palliative care as *nurturing.* There is a very necessary need for comfort and compassion when one is recovering from a period of cancer diagnosis and treatment, and the whole saga of being a patient. I say saga because I feel it needs to be highlighted that for someone who is recovering and in an ongoing fatigue state, whatever the original or subsequent cause, every blood test, clinic visit, GP visit and treatment session can be felt as a hardship, even if it is provided by thoughtful, experienced, professional and highly competent practitioners. Routine tasks like finding a car parking spot or having to wait a long time to be seen by a doctor or nurse practitioner can add to feeling exhausted. This exhaustion or fatigue is often accompanied by less welcomed emotions such as sadness, depression, anger or non-specific anxiety which only add to the struggle to stay awake and function. After months of being in the 'sick role' as coined by Talcott Parsons, the medical sociologist, the physical and emotional fields of the body are depleted and weakened, that is, muscles are reduced in size and function; confidence and self-efficacy is lessened; hypersensitivity to the external environment is increased and mental acuity can also be affected negatively. The internal energy resources used to get through months or years of treatment protocols may have worn out. With all this going on for so long, and now acknowledged and understood, there is an imperative for restoration and invigoration. At the top of the list for many people and a priority for most is the need for refuelling, restocking and replenishment—nourishment, nurturance, comfort and even some indulgence to bring back the unique and most valued whole and 'invincible self' that may have been lost.

When thinking of nourishment, we tend to turn our attention to nutrients and calories, which are crucial of course, particularly when recovering from energy-zapping cancer treatments of surgery, chemotherapy and radiotherapy. In addition, the emotional burden of a cancer diagnosis comes with deep stress that is often internalised. The associated hyper-arousal of the limbic area of the brain can be harmful as it interferes with joyful and productive endeavours. Vitamins, minerals, micronutrients, superfoods, proteins, healthy fats, complex carbohydrates and clean water are all critical to the body's ability to repair, rejuvenate and strengthen and to our mental and cognitive health (Rucklidge et al. 2021). A conscious, varied and balanced diet of whole foods grown on nutrient-rich, preferably certified organic soil, transported with respect and delivered in good quality condition will promote health and wellness in contrast to a diet consisting of heavily processed and packaged products that hardly deserve to be called food. Sustenance from non-plant sources of nutrition such as lean meats and fish are excellent too, provided they are not full of antibiotics, artificial hormones, and harmful toxic contaminants such as pesticides and insecticides.

Our mental, emotional and spiritual well-being is also fundamental to our health, whatever our circumstances or beliefs. If we consider nourishment in a broader context that affects all of our senses, then we can tap into our creative and artistic selves and find nourishment in our surroundings. There is nourishment to be absorbed from all kinds of nature, whether you are near the sea, woodland, mountains, grasslands, garden or city park; or the kind, thoughtful generousity of humanity; or touching and being touched by deliciously sumptuous fabrics; or an interesting book or program that nourishes your intellect and thought processes or enchanting music that matches your mood or preference at a specific moment. The list can go on and on of course. The point is that we can find nourishment in so many ways beyond what we ingest. The emphasis here is sustaining and supporting the vital functions of the body and also the mind and spirit. Nutritionally we require a balanced diet that provides the essential components to enable the intricacies of the biochemical interactions to occur. These include the complex processes of the hormonal and neurological networks, digestion and muscle functioning.

However, as human beings, we are more than our physical bodies. I have struggled to decide in the context of the Energy Restorative Framework whether *nourishment* or *nurturance* should be used as a core concept and attribute. In analysing the early studies, nurturing activities emerged, however, nourishment seemed to go wider and be more comprehensive. I was drawing on my perceptions and also discussions with the people that surrounded me. I finally decided to succumb to doing some internet research and found out that both words come from the Latin verb *nutrire*, which means to suckle or to nourish a child or someone in need of support and care.

From dictionary sources I discovered that nurturance could mean:

- Affectionate care and attention.
- Emotional and physical nourishment and care given to someone as in 'sources of nurturance and security.'
- The act of encouraging, nourishing and caring for someone.

Also, *affective nurturance* refers to meeting an individual's emotional needs. That is interesting.

From dictionary sources, nurture can mean:
- To take care of, referring to feed or protect, as you would in reference to children or plants.

So, nurturing can mean being cared for and looked after and also a quality that provides encouragement and acceptance of oneself. Therapeutically, this is the aspect of the attribute that I wish to emphasise for the person who is troubled by fatigue. As a healthcare professional we can recognise the value of providing individualised support under the banner of nurturance and nourishment. It is back to asking: What does the person require now? Is it nutritional nourishment? A feeling of safety and acceptance? A sensuous and considerate lover? A luxurious massage with soothing essential oils? Or perhaps encouragement to follow a lifelong dream to unlock their creative self?

References

Aron AP, Aron EN. Love and the expansion of self: understanding attraction and satisfaction. Washington, DC: Hemisphere; 1986.

Baird J. Phosphorescence. On awe, wonder and things that sustain you when the world goes dark. Sydney: Fourth Estate. HarperCollins Publishers Australia; 2020.

Bandura A. Self-efficacy: toward a unifying theory of behavioral change. Psychol Rev. 1977;84(2):191–215.

Dys-Steenbergen O, Wright SC, Aron A. Self-expansion motivation improves cross-group interactions and enhances self-growth. Group Process Intergroup Relat. 2016;19(1):60–71. https://doi.org/10.1177/1368430215583517.

Ennis G, Kirshbaum MN, Waheed N. The beneficial attributes of visual art- making in cancer care: an integrative review. Eur J Cancer Care. 2017;29:71–8. https://doi.org/10.1111/ecc.12663.

Ennis G, Kirshbaum M, Waheed N. The energy-enhancing potential of participatory performance-based arts activities in the care of people with a diagnosis of cancer: an integrative review. Arts Health. 2019;11(2):87–103. https://doi.org/10.1080/17533015.2018.1443951.

Garner BA. Garner's modern English usage. Oxford: Oxford University Press; 2016.

Kaplan S. The restorative benefits of nature: toward an integrative framework. J Environ Psychol. 1995;15:169–82.

Kaplan S. Meditation, restoration and the management of mental fatigue. Environ Behav. 2001;33:480–506.

Kirshbaum M, Ennis G, Waheed N. Art in cancer care: exploring the role of visual art-making programs within an energy restoration framework. Eur J Oncol Nurs. 2017;29:71–8. https://doi.org/10.1016/j.ejon.2017.05.003.

Mattingly B, Lewandowski G. An expanded self is a more capable self: the association between self-concept size and self-efficacy. Self Identity. 2013;12(6):621–34. https://doi.org/10.108 0/15298868.2012.718863.

Mattingly BA, Lewandowski GW. Broadening horizons: self-expansion in relational and non-relational contexts. Soc Personal Psychol Compass. 2014;8(1):30–40. https://doi.org/10.1111/ spc3.12080.

Rucklidge JJ, Johnstone JM, Kaplan BJ. Nutrition provides the essential foundation for optimizing mental health. Evid Based Pract Child Adolescent Mental Health. 2021;6(1):131–54. https:// doi.org/10.1080/23794925.2021.1875342.

Turner T-p. Belonging, remembering ourselves home. In: Her Own Room Press; 2017.

Wilson C. Designing the purposeful organization: how to inspire business performance beyond boundaries, 1st ed. Kogan Page; 2015. http://search.ebscohost.com/login.aspx?direct=true&A uthType=shib&db=e000xww&AN=944498&site=ehost-live

The Joyful Freedom Approach

10

10.1 Introduction

Throughout my professional life spanning three continents, I have known and continue to observe many people who suffer from diagnosed chronic and acute illnesses and conditions; numbing fear; brutal and economic hardships; cruel and destructive relationships; severe reactive sadness and despair; and imposed, disrespectful limitations that stifle natural curiosity and creative expression. These situations represent only the 'tip of the iceberg' that has resulted in a global epidemic of people who feel and are noticeably sick, in pain, hurt, traumatised, angry, fearful, resentful, frustrated, impotent, disgraced, denigrated, depressed, anxious, ashamed, helpless, lethargic, fatigued and completely exhausted! Wow. This is a sorry realisation that left me to contemplate and ask: Where is the joy in the world? (Fig. 10.1) Where is the child-like joy in people's lives? Where has it gone? Would a focus on joy be useful to aid healing and promote health and well-being for all? Could this seemingly simplistic perspective make a difference? Well, I decided to take this on, particularly as I knew cognitively that it aligned well with the research in cancer-related fatigue that has held my attention for so long.

So, what is joy? Before I searched the literature, my view of joy was as another one of those subjective sentiments, emotions or reactions to internal and external stimuli, such as anger, guilt, pain, anxiety and shame that seemed to flow through the body and psyche involuntarily. Yet, after sitting a bit longer in thought, I realised that joy is quite different; it is pure when it is experienced and deliciously desired. We unconsciously yearn for it and may fall into despair and hopelessness when we realise that it is not part of our lives anymore. Furthermore, joy comes from within often as an internal, secret smile accompanied by happy energy that can be declared exuberantly as in the children's song:

> *[Everybody sing:] If you're happy and you know it clap your hands, if you're happy and you know it clap your hands, if you're happy and you know it and you really want to show it, if you're happy and you know it clap your hands ....*

© Springer Nature Switzerland AG 2021
M. N. Kirshbaum, *The Joyful Freedom Approach to Cancer-Related Fatigue*,
https://doi.org/10.1007/978-3-030-76932-1_10

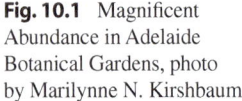

Fig. 10.1 Magnificent
Abundance in Adelaide
Botanical Gardens, photo
by Marilynne N. Kirshbaum

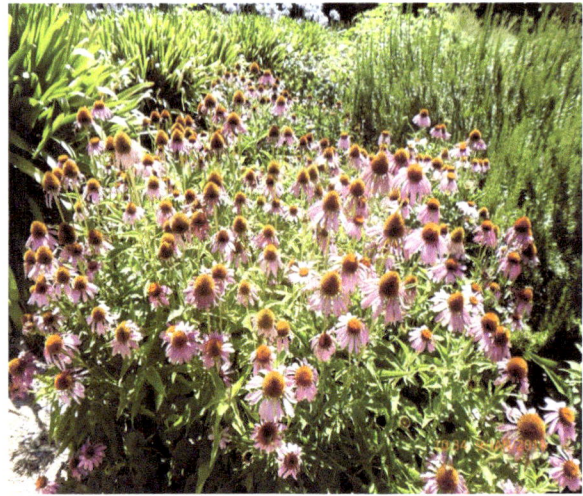

Joy is also authentic, personal, child-like and can be peaceful and exuberant at the same time!

But if this is so desirable and pleasant, what stands in the way of experiencing this emotion as often as possible? I did not have to think too long for words to pop up that described day-to day life as characterised by a conglomerate of worries, constraints, burdens, pain and [oh dear,] oppression. Then, it occurred to me spontaneously that freedom, as a state of longing, brought up so many positive examples of how it could make a positive impact on aspects of wellbeing and… move us closer to joy! For example, having the freedom to live as you please (without shame or disgrace), to dress as you want (without feeling criticized or self-conscious), to spend the day according to your whims (without compromise), to feel the ease of breathing fully and deeply (without fear, obstruction or pollution) and to find the freedom to explore and experiment to discover what you truly enjoy doing. This last 'freedom' and guidance of how to bring in and access the life-force quality of highly motivational energy that best supports, stimulates and enlivens the person is what stands out for me. That is why it is the cornerstone of the Joyful Freedom Approach to Energy Restoration and the personally motivating inspiration for this unique book.

The Joyful Freedom Approach is a program of recovery from energy depletion caused by any distressing life event such as illness, surgery or separation. The approach is aimed at helping people to discover what they can do to energise their lives following an event that has left them lacking vitality, wellness or a sense of direction and clarity about how to live life fully and joyfully. The approach, aligned to the emergent Energy Restoration Theory and Framework, has been developed over many years from a background of cancer nursing, counselling, hypnotherapy, Reiki, shamanic journeying, sacred sexual healing and art-based experiences.

The Joyful Freedom Approach offers practical, integral and integrated guidance to improve mental, emotional, spiritual, sexual and physical health. The approach is gentle, caring-based and flexible as it draws on the unique gifts, talents and preferences of people to release and unblock whatever is holding them back from living life to its fullest. Each individual iteration of the program is designed with compassion and love to promote the flow of energy and creativity and is intended to be expansive, creative, fun, powerful, empowering and meaningful to the individual.

This unique approach can be viewed as a salve for living in a world full of uncertainty, struggle and disaster; it can bring calm and creativity into one's precious life and help us all to break free from the suppression and repression of distressful events often experienced as lethargy, sadness, pain, inertia, frustration or worry.

The actual program has been developed to take place over six sessions, excluding follow-ups. There is a stepwise structure and plan for the type of intervention activity for each session; however, the program can be adapted to suit the character and therapeutic modalities of the particular practitioner or counsellor. Ideally, the sessions are weekly or biweekly; however, the frequency is dependent upon the preferences of the client and practitioner.

The sessions are planned to follow the guiding structure:

1. Relax, ground and centre
2. Reveal and meet yourself
3. Release the blocks that stand in your way
4. Restore yourself to optimum joy and freedom
5. Finalisation of the Toolkit of Expressions and Energy Restoration Plan
6. Review
   (a) Follow-up sessions as required or requested

The program begins with asking the client to identify the problem and proceeds to offer opportunities to *relax, ground and centre*. This will help in-depth discussions about personal history and biography. The client is asked to write a journal with prompts to identify significant moments in their life and asked to share only parts with the practitioner. The journal writing is an important part of *reveal and meet yourself.* Within these two early sessions, the attributes of the Energy Restorative Framework, *Purposeful, Expanding, Connecting, Awe-inspiring and Nourishing,* are explained. There is also an exploration around the client's usual strategies of coping when tired or lethargic. The opportunity to experiment with different activities and pursuits is presented, which will be the focus of the rest of the program session. Meanwhile, a list of restorative activities (the **Expressions**, see Table 9.1) that fall under each attribute category is formulated; this will be a useful dynamic toolkit that can be reviewed and adapted for many years to come. An Energy Restoration Plan is an action plan that is developed where identified challenges such as blocks, attachments, fears and tensions are delineated and thoughtfully addressed through small, achievable objectives.

The program is intended to be used creatively—and to home in on the qualities of expansiveness and fascination within a safe and nourishing therapeutic environment. I have piloted and evaluated the program on a small cohort of volunteer clients so far. All have benefited from the highly individualised and quite novel approach.

10.2   Future Horizons

As part of the Joyful Freedom Approach, a host of interventions, treatments and pursuits can be incorporated into an individualised program. This depends on the skillset and character of the practitioner and the willingness and interest of the client to try something new. For example, just to name a few options: hypnotherapy, energy healing, breathwork [many kinds], remedial bodywork, somatic bodywork, spiritual healing, shamanic journeying, sexual shamanic healing, soul contract reading, crystal healing, Akashic record reading, transpersonal psychotherapy, evolutionary astrology and plant medicine might all be beneficial to the person who experiences fatigue and lethargy. Each of these examples will potentially enable an individual to break through limitations and make beneficial changes to their lives. Possibly. Most probably. It is beyond the scope of this book to address and evaluate each of the infinite offerings of alternative practitioners and coaches. However, I would like to emphasise the importance and value to you, as a healthcare practitioner, of exploration and experimentation across all the attributes, elements and domains—in a range of ways. If you feel like your energy and your life is stuck then you will need to decide what you can do to create a shift, even a small one. From your experiences, you can consider passing on, even just the aspect of being openminded, to your clients and patients. So, my advice to everyone, health care practitioners, their clients and freeagents is to try out different pursuits and develop a dynamic action plan—even if some of the pursuits may seem a bit 'wacky' and not included in credible guidelines or a Cochrane Review, yet. Why not try something new? Test it out for yourself. Write about it and share it with the world. As I have said before, there is plenty of work to be done. I truly wish you all the very best that life has to offer.

To Joyful Freedom for All

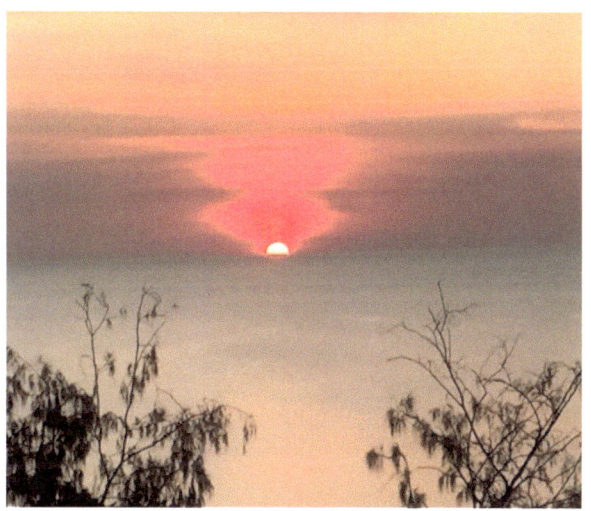

© Springer Nature Switzerland AG 2021   131
M. N. Kirshbaum, *The Joyful Freedom Approach to Cancer-Related Fatigue*,
https://doi.org/10.1007/978-3-030-76932-1

Relevant Publications by Same Author

Ennis G, Kirshbaum MN, Waheed N. The beneficial attributes of visual art-making in cancer care: an integrative review. Eur J Cancer Care. 2017;27(1) https://doi.org/10.1111/ecc.12663.

Ennis GM, Kirshbaum M, Waheed N. The energy-enhancing potential of participatory performance-based arts activities in the care of people with a diagnosis of cancer: an integrative review. Arts Health. 2018; https://doi.org/10.1080/17533015.2018.1443951.

Kirshbaum M. Lymphoedema massage: a valued nursing intervention. Prof Nurse. 1996;11(4): 230–2.

Kirshbaum M. Neutropenia: more than a low neutrophil count. Eur J Oncol Nurs. 1998;2(2):115–22.

Kirshbaum M. Lymphoedema and breast cancer. Nursing Times Clinical Monograph No 38. London: Emap Healthcare; 1999.

Kirshbaum M. Promoting physical exercise in breast cancer care. Nurs Stand. 2005;19(41):41–8. https://doi.org/10.7748/ns.19.41.41.s52.

Kirshbaum M. A review of the benefits of whole body exercise during and after treatment for breast cancer. J Clin Nurs. 2007;6(1):104–21. https://doi.org/10.1111/j.1365-2702.2006.01638.x.

Kirshbaum M. Translation to practice: a RCT of an evidenced based booklet targeted at breast care nurses in Britain. Worldviews Evid Based Nurs. 2008;5(2):60–74. https://doi.org/10.1111/j.1741-6787.2008.00113.x.

Kirshbaum M. Cancer related fatigue: a review of nursing interventions. Br J Community Nurs. 2010;15(5):220–4. https://doi.org/10.12968/bjcn.2010.15.5.47945.

Kirshbaum M. Pharmacological treatments for fatigue associated with palliative care. Clin J Oncol Nurs. 2011;15(4):438–9. https://doi.org/10.1188/11.CJON.438-439.

Kirshbaum M. Cochrane review brief: exercise interventions on health-related quality of life for cancer survivors. OJIN. 2013;18(3)

Kirshbaum M, Donbavand J. Making the most out of life: exploring the contribution of attention restorative theory in developing a non pharmacological intervention for fatigue. Palliat Support Care. 2014;12(6):473–80. https://doi.org/10.1017/S1478951513000539.

Kirshbaum M, Olson K, Pongthavornkamol K, Graffigna G. Understanding the meaning of fatigue at the end of life: an ethnoscience study. Eur J Oncol Nurs. 2013;17:146–53. https://doi.org/10.1016/j.ejon.2012.04.007.

Kirshbaum MN, Stead M, Bartys S. An exploratory study of Reiki experiences in women who have cancer. Int J Palliat Nurs. 2016;22(4):166–72. https://doi.org/10.12968/ijpn.2016.22.4.166.

Kirshbaum M, Ennis G, Waheed N. Art in cancer care: exploring the role of visual art-making programs within an energy restoration framework. Eur J Oncol Nurs. 2017;29:71–8. https://doi.org/10.1016/j.ejon.2017.05.003.

© Springer Nature Switzerland AG 2021
M. N. Kirshbaum, *The Joyful Freedom Approach to Cancer-Related Fatigue*,
https://doi.org/10.1007/978-3-030-76932-1